THE WAY OF WISDOM FOR HEALTH:

Optimism, Kindness, Motivation, Movement, Nutrition, Stress Control and 17 Wise Ways to Outsmart Diabetes on a Daily Basis

KEN ELLIS, M.S.
with Deb Ellis

DISCLAIMER: The information in this book should
not replace consultations with qualified health care
professionals to meet your individual medical needs.

Also by Ken Ellis

The Way of Wisdom for Diabetes:
Cope with Stress, Move More, Lose Weight
and Keep Hope Alive

Subscribe to the
"Wisdom, Good News, Health and Wellness"
newsletter at
www.wisdomfordiabetes.org

Thank You...

To Max, my brother who has been such an encouragement
to me and has encouraged thousands of students as a caring
professor of Mathematics and Campus Minister for decades.

To my dear sister, Janice, whose kindness to family
and friends also extends to many participants in
Weight Watchers and has for many years!

—Ken

Contents

THE POWER
FOR HEALTH
AND WELLNESS

INTRODUCTION

The Power of Wisdom

"Do not let them out of your sight, keep them within your heart; for they are life to those who find them and health to one's whole body...The wise prevail through great power, and those who have knowledge muster their strength" (Proverbs 4:21-22, 24:5).

E veryone wants to have a loving family, be healthy, be wise, get along with others, or be admired, don't they? Doesn't everyone want to change, improve, or get better? Now we are really getting to the crux of the matter...James Irwin an astronaut of the Apollo 15 mission (July 30, 1971), that landed on the moon presumably had this to say about change "You might think going to the moon was the most scientific project ever, but they literally 'threw us' in the direction of the moon. We had to adjust our course every ten minutes and landed only fifty feet inside of the 500-mile radius of our target." On that mission, every change, no matter how small, was essential to success. Barriers, obstacles or roadblocks have to be removed or broken through to change. Habits can be barriers. When we get in a routine it becomes a habit. Horace Mann said, "Habits are like a cable. We weave a strand of it every day, and soon it cannot be broken." It takes a different way of thinking, a new attitude to improve or change.

Is everyone's attitude like that of a veteran who learns to read at age eighty-nine? "Toughest thing that ever happened to me in my life is not being able to read," Ed Bray said. He's an eighty-nine-year old World War II veteran who just read his first book. Remarkable is his story for what he accomplished—a decorated World War II veteran, D-day survivor, awarded two Purple Hearts—without ever learning to read. He is learning to read now at the Wadley Reading and Technology Center at Northeastern State University, Tahlequah, OK. Most that come are in grade school. The director of the reading center, Dr. Tobi Thompson said, "It's rare to find an adult who has made it nine decades without learning how to read. She adds that "his story is an inspiration for anyone who questions whether it's too late to learn." "His quote that is now all over NSU is, 'Get in there and learn, baby, now, because you're not going to learn in that pine box,' and that's something that I think we all need to take to heart," Thompson said.[1] Watch "WWII veteran refuses to close the book on his life" at https://www.youtube.com/watch?v=MczEU0QAJ-E

Again, doesn't everyone want to change, improve, or get better? Doesn't everyone want to live a longer life? Doesn't everyone want to live the good life? No, because the attitude of many is just give me a pill or three easy steps to health and wellness so that I don't have to change. So often we have to change our attitudes in order to get the best results. The following story will help give you some background on why I feel a deep concern for those with chronic diseases like diabetes. Change is needed when people are diagnosed with diabetes or any chronic disease. Denial, living the way they've always lived without any changes can lead to the harm of their health! I don't want that to happen. Since you are reading this I believe you don't want that to happen either. The story is told of a little second-grade boy who was trying out for a part in the school play. The day came for the auditions and his mother took him to school and waited for him to come out. She was nervous because she knew he couldn't sing, couldn't act, and couldn't memorize very well. So, she was surprised when he came out after forty-five minutes with a big smile on his face. "How did it go, honey?" "It was great, Mom. Guess what? I've been chosen to clap and cheer." Not that I've been chosen to "clap and cheer" or encourage those with diabetes and chronic diseases, but I'm choosing to do so! One reason is because I've discovered the powerful teachings of wisdom found in the book of Proverbs to be so helpful, bringing hope and encouragement! I want us all to experience that encouragement!

When I was diagnosed on December 20, 1960, with Type 1 Diabetes, I was in the first grade, and the little word diabetes had such an impact on my dad that he became lightheaded and almost passed out. That type of reaction is not unique but has been repeated numerous times by other parents of children with diabetes. For example, watch "Diabetes Fears" at https://www.

youtube.com/watch?v=MPWjJ2OdN1A. Any one, however, who hears the words "You have diabetes," whether it is Type 1 or Type 2, will be hearing three words he or she doesn't want to hear. The same could be said of "heart disease, cancer, lupus, rheumatoid arthritis, multiple sclerosis!"

Challenges confront our sense of well-being. Hope is needed! The Proverbs are short pithy sayings of wisdom and wisdom brings hope for every area of life. Wisdom is the skill for living. *"A good person gives life to others; **the wise person teaches others how to live"** (Proverbs 11:30 NCV). One important area of our lives is our health. These wisdom teachings from the book of Proverbs bring health and wellness. *"My son, pay attention to what I say; turn your ear to my words. Do not let them out of your sight, keep them within your heart; for they are life to those who find them and health to one's whole body"* (Proverbs 4:20-22).

Our attitude makes the difference. *"The spirit of a man will sustain him in sickness, but who can bear a broken spirit?"* (Proverbs 18:14 NKJV) or *"The will to live can get you through sickness, but no one can live with a broken spirit"* (Proverbs 18:14 NCV). Optimism, hopefulness, cheerfulness and confidence are the benefits of the way of wisdom.

An optimistic attitude is a strength that combats health challenges and contributes to a measure of wellness! We need motivation, tools and resources to help. In this book I will show how God cares about you as seen in his wisdom. You will read of his wisdom being applied in various situations. Consider this proverb. *"Trust in the Lord with all your heart, and do not rely on your own insight. In all your ways acknowledge him, and he will make straight your paths"* (Proverbs 3:5-6). "Trust" is a concept that includes the idea of safety, confidence, and security. A sense of security and safety come by following God's way or wisdom. Using the principles of God's wisdom is like preparations for a road, removing obstacles, smoothing and leveling the path. By using his wisdom life becomes straight, bringing safety, confidence, and better health. This will apply to every area of life since he said for us to acknowledge him in all of our ways.

Learning to acknowledge God and his wisdom in a wide variety of different situations gives us hope and success. Does the following statement motivate you? *"For the LORD gives wisdom; from his mouth come knowledge and understanding. He holds success (or victory) in store for the upright"* (Proverbs 2:7-8). Success is motivational; it helps us focus on a goal. And God gives his wisdom for us to succeed, to have victory in life. God cares about us! His wisdom blesses us! *"Blessed are those who find wisdom, those who gain understanding"* (Proverbs 3:13). Here are some examples of very helpful "way of wisdom" principles:

HOPE

"Hope in the future brings strength to the present."

"Eat honey, my son, for it is good; honey from the comb is sweet to your taste. Know also that wisdom is like honey for you: If you find it, there is a future hope for you, and your hope will not be cut off." (Proverbs 24:13-14).

The news media touts one possible cure after another for diabetes. They've been doing this for years while I continue to live with the disease one decade after another. Yes, it was a big day when actual blood glucose could be checked at home with a meter rather than go to a lab. I lived more than twenty years with diabetes before that significant change took place, getting my first glucose meter in 1981.

Research has brought more innovative devices that keep improving like insulin pumps and now continuous glucose monitors. Research is introducing on the market now a "hybrid closed-loop (HCL)" system where the continuous glucose sensors will work with the insulin pump to automatically release or slow the release of insulin (only the basal dose, not the bolus for meals. The bolus still has to be done manually.), depending on the glucose levels. Now it has to be done manually by the person wearing the pump.[2] In the future beta cell transplants may be done with approximately 150 million cells that would have to be transplanted into each patient being treated.[3] Beta cells produce insulin in a multistep process.

Even though this sounds exciting, neither you nor I can just sit back with anticipation and wait for their arrival. We have to continue to live our lives day in and day out. Another factor we all need to consider is how expensive these innovations as well as new medications are. That's why God's wisdom is so beneficial, giving us hope to cope each day. We are rewarded by using the "the way of wisdom" principles. We don't have to wait for them. They're already available! *"For through wisdom your days will be many, and years will be added to your life. If you are wise, your wisdom will reward you"* (Proverbs 9:11-12). Here is another wisdom principle to use:

MAKE PLANS

"It pays to plan ahead. It wasn't raining when Noah built the ark. (More than a hundred years later it rained.)"

Diligence is associated with planning in the following passages: *"The lazy do not roast any game, but the diligent feed on the riches of the hunt"* (Proverbs 12:27). *"The plans of the diligent lead to profit as sure as haste leads to poverty"* (Proverbs 21:5). Another way to word this is, "The plans of the planner lead to profit." Diligence is used in several Bible passages with the idea of cut, quick and decisive, or determined before the situation arises. Something that is cut cannot be uncut. The decision is made ahead of time, and thus what to do can be determined quickly, because the decision has already been made before the situation arises. No distraction would carry the person off course. (Read 2 Samuel 5:23–24 and 1 Kings 20:40 for more examples of the use of the word diligence. In 2 Samuel 5:24 the word is translated "move quickly" or "act promptly" or "act decisively" because the decision has already been made.)

The concept of diligence is described in the following proverbs: *"The sluggard craves and gets nothing, but the desires of the diligent are fully satisfied"* (Proverbs 13:4). *"Sluggards do not plow in season; so, at harvest time they look but find nothing"* (Proverbs 20: 4). The word "satisfied" in Proverbs 13:4 could also be translated "prosper" like it is in Proverbs 11:25. It means "to be fat, grow fat, become fat, become prosperous." In other words, in contrast to skin and bones, healthy is what it means. Diligence, according to the way of wisdom, is actually the "decide ahead of time" principle, which brings health.

So why is this wisdom principle so helpful? Planning ahead makes the difference. You may already use this principle with your medication. When you fill your "7 Day AM/PM Pill Container" that is diligence, that is planning ahead. Forgetting a pill is not good! I use this principle for my oral medications. How many steps will you take today? How many carbohydrates will you eat? How many times will you check your blood glucose today? Will you check your blood pressure? Will you record your blood glucose, blood pressure, steps, calories, carbohydrates? This is all diligence, planning ahead. Start doing this. Diligence, planning ahead will give us more confidence and a better sense of control.

MINDFUL VERSUS MINDLESS THINKING

"It is just a thought, but it could change your life."

"What you think doesn't really count." Is that true? Read the following words and see if they count. *"Blessed are those who find wisdom, those who gain understanding, for she is more profitable than silver and yields better returns than gold. She is more precious than rubies; nothing you desire can compare with her. Long life is in her right hand; in her left hand are riches and honor. Her ways are pleasant ways, and all her paths are peace. She is a tree of life to those who take hold of her; those who hold her fast will be blessed... Listen, my son, accept what I say, and the years of your life will be many"* (Proverbs 3:13-18, 4:10). To me those words count; they are positive, uplifting words that build my confidence and give me hope. *"Be careful what you think, because your thoughts run your life"* (Proverbs 4:23 NCV).

Can you really resist any temptation like candy, cookies and pastries that are seen on the counter or desk? In sight in mind and what is in mind brings actions like yielding to temptations. Dr. Wansink has researched what happens when candy dishes are easily seen and accessible.[4] He concludes from his research that when food is out of sight, it is out of mind. When administrative assistants saw the candy on their desks they ate seventy-four more calories of the candy than when it was hidden in their desks. When the candy is shouting in your face, grabbing your attention, tempting you to grab one then it is easily done! Looking at the candy, the candy is in mind and then eaten. So, the wisdom teaching comes true—*"Be careful what you think, because your thoughts run your life"* (Proverbs 4:23).

PERSISTENCE

"The man of the hour spent many days and nights getting there. Remember, overnight success takes about ten years."

I've checked my blood glucose more the 100,000 times. It wasn't all done in a week, month or year, but rather more than thirty-seven years, one prick at a time. In 1981 the first glucose meters became available. That is when I got my Ames meter, a very cumbersome meter to use, taking a large drop of blood and two minutes to get the blood glucose result. Persistence in checking my blood glucose has been an important key to my health.

Without doing this I couldn't make corrections with insulin if blood glucose was elevated. People with diabetes need to consistently and persistently check their blood glucose so that corrections can be made if the blood glucose is elevated. Corrections like not eating carbohydrates for the next meal, delaying the meal, taking a leisure walk before the meal or for those using insulin a correction dose. Not giving up makes the difference for health and well-being. Consider the following...

"The trouble with most people is that they stop trying in trying times. Trying times are no time to quit trying. Keep trying when others quit." Vince Lombardi said, "Once you learn to quit, it becomes a habit." Paul J. Meyer wrote, "Ninety percent of those who fail are not actually defeated. They simply quit." Discouragement can easily come when you don't feel good. We all face discouraging times especially with our own health or with the health of someone we love. So, the question is "are we going to give up or get up?" God with his wisdom encourages us to get up! *"A good person gives life to others; the wise person teaches others how to live...Doing evil brings no safety at all, but a good person has safety and security...The wicked want what other evil people have stolen, but good people want to give what they have to others...Don't be wicked and attack a good family's house; don't rob the place where they live. Even though good people may be bothered by trouble seven times, they are never defeated, but the wicked are overwhelmed by trouble"* (Proverbs 11:30, 12:3, 12:12, 24:15-16 NCV).

EMPATHY

People who live for themselves are in a mighty small business. Lift people up, don't put people down.

Encouragement makes a difference in the lives of the encourager and the encouraged. How can we be encouraging to others; how can we lift them up?

When Napoleon and his army invaded Russia in 1812, the story goes that he was separated from his men in a small town. His enemy saw him, pursuing him through the winding streets of the town. Running for his life, he ducked into a furrier's shop. Gasping for breath, he begged the man to hide him, saying, "Save me, save me!" "Where can I hide?" He covered him under a big pile of furs in the corner. Suddenly the door was thrown open and the Russians shouted, "Where is he?" Over his protests, they began tearing his shop apart in search of Napoleon. When they came to the pile of furs, poking it with their swords, they amazingly missed him so they left.

As Napoleon cautiously uncovered himself his personal guards entered the shop. The owner of the shop knew Napoleon was almost killed, coming out of the pile of furs untouched by any blade. Wondering how Napoleon felt during that horrifying time, he asked him "What was it like being under those furs, knowing that any second could be your last?

Outraged by such a question, Napoleon stood up to his full 5'7" height, telling his guards to take this insolent man out, blindfold him and execute him. "I will personally give the command to fire myself!" Blindfolding him and dragging him outside, they stood him before a wall. Seeing nothing, but hearing the guards shuffling in place preparing their rifles, tears began to pour down his face in abject fear! Napoleon shouted "Ready, aim!" The man was terrified.

Instead of hearing guns firing he heard the blindfold being torn from his face. With the sun glaring in his face he saw Napoleon staring into his eyes. Then Napoleon said, "Now you know!"

That story reminds me of the life of Job and his so-called friend Eliphaz. He thought he knew more than he actually did when he said to Job: *"What do you know that we don't know? What insights do you have that we don't have?"* (Job 15:9) Here is Eliphaz, healthy, wealthy, and wise, talking to his friend who has just lost all ten of his grown children in what sounds like a tornado. Job's grieving wife has been driven to despair; his health is now gone, replaced with excruciating pain; and his status in life is completely changed with the loss of his wealth, the loss of just about everything he has; and he now feels alienated from God. And now this wealthy, healthy, wise man, Eliphaz, asks, *"What do you know that we don't know?"* Do you get the picture? What Eliphaz does not know is called experience—Job's excruciating pain and loss!

"Fools find no pleasure in understanding but delight in airing their own opinions" (Proverbs 18:2). That proverb describes Eliphaz. Understanding and kindness go together and benefit the one in need. The way of wisdom teaches us to be kind to the needy. *"Blessed is the one who is kind to the needy"* (Proverbs 14:21). *"The one who gets wisdom loves life; the one who cherishes understanding will soon prosper"* (Proverbs 19:8). The way of wisdom teaches that happiness results from being kind and being

understanding brings prosperity or wellness. There is a great contrast between understanding words and judgmental words. Which would you rather hear from the following examples: "You shouldn't dwell on the negative" or "It's hard to find anything good at times like this, isn't it?" "Don't you know it could always be worse?" Or "It probably seems very overwhelming right now to you." "You've got to keep smiling and looking for the positive" or "I'm impressed that you're able to keep going."[5] We need to strive to be understanding because no one can say "I know exactly how you feel." *"Each heart knows its own sadness. And no one else can share its joy"* (Proverbs 14:10). *"A kindhearted woman gains honor, but ruthless men gain only wealth. Those who are kind benefit themselves, but the cruel bring ruin on themselves... A generous person will prosper; whoever refreshes others will be refreshed"* (Proverbs 11:16-17, 25).

God's wisdom is relevant for every area of our lives!

The major change for us to have is to see how relevant God's wisdom is in every area of our lives, including our health. The good news is we can use it. *"Through wisdom your days will be many, and years will be added to your life. If you are wise, your wisdom will reward you"* (Proverbs 9:11-12). This is a wonderful resource that God is providing for our use! We'll examine a health concern at the beginning of each chapter and then examples of how wisdom applies to related situations. At the end of each chapter relevant applications or "health prescriptions" will be made of wisdom for our health. We'll examine how these wisdom teachings apply to movement or exercise, meal planning or nutrition, motivation, kindness or helping others, controlling stress and building an optimistic attitude. In the last three chapters, I will show how I've used wisdom to manage my diabetes for most of my life—almost sixty years with diabetes. You will see seventeen ways to outsmart diabetes on a daily basis! As an introduction, consider how wisdom applies to the following examples of a sixteen-year old whose arm was lost in a shark attack, a seventeen-year old overcoming cancer, literal storms we face, people hearing for the first time and a man painting an elderly neighbor's house.

SHARK ATTACK

"Things turn out best for those who make the best out of the way that things turn out."

Several weeks ago, I began to ponder this intriguing proverb. *"The fear of the LORD leads to life: Then one rests content, untouched by trouble"* (Proverbs 19:23). What does he mean untouched by trouble? Everyone encounters trouble. Just living, interacting with the choices that others make can bring about trouble. When strong forces of wind hit a tree, the tree can remain intact, in a sense untouched by the storm. This happens if its root system is strong. Isn't that what the proverb is saying about the fear of the Lord as our root system? Paul, when writing to the church at Philippi, said, *"But one thing I do: Forgetting what is behind and straining toward what is ahead, I press on toward the goal to win the prize for which God has called me heavenward in Christ Jesus"* (Philippians 3:13-14). It wasn't that Paul couldn't remember what he had done in the past, but that he was not going to let the past dictate his decisions for the present. Thus, he was living untouched by the troubles he caused in the past, persecuting Christians.

Tragedy of various kinds strikes people either leaving them deeply troubled and unable to function or leaves them untouched because they have the attitude to cope. It has been said "Things turn out best for those who make the best out of the way that things turn out." Making the best, being untouched, making the best decisions out of tragedy was profoundly demonstrated in a sixteen-year old recently who survived a shark attack.[6] He lost his left arm while he was waist deep in water on a beach in North Carolina. "We were just playing around in the waves, and I felt a hit on my left calf," he said. "I thought it felt like a big fish, and I started moving away. And then the shark bit my arm—off." "That was the first time I saw it, when it was biting up my left arm," he said.

As he is being interviewed in his hospital bed recovering from the shock of what happened, he said something very profound and wise for a sixteen-year old. "I have two options: I can try to live my life the way I was and make an effort to do that even though I don't have an arm, or I can just let this be completely debilitating and bring my life down and ruin it," Hunter Treschl said. "Out of those two, there's really only one that I would actually choose and that's to try to fight and live a normal life with the cards I've been dealt." I don't know if he has ever heard of the proverb we are discussing or if he fears the Lord, but that is the kind of attitude we should also have, having the respect of the Lord. Let's make a conscious effort, in the days to come, to respect the Lord more and more so that the proverb will come true for us when tragedy confronts us! You can view the interview with Hunter at https://www.youtube.com/watch?v=OuJkkVZW_FI

A TEEN, A PUPPY, A SMILE AND GOD'S WISDOM

"One smile can't change the world, but
your smile changes mine."

It seems the news media reports the bad news to the exclusion of the good news. Occasionally, the good news breaks through the endless barrier of bad news. It recently happened with the story of an English bulldog puppy. By changing our focus from a life-threatening illness for seventeen-year old Storm Miller to a good news story, it gives a sense of revival.[7] Last January he was diagnosed with a form of cancer called "Synovial Cell Sarcoma." Storm made a wish for a puppy and his wish came true by the Make-A-Wish®Michigan organization. (Their purpose is to grant about one wish per day for a child with a life-threatening medical condition).

The day he had anticipated of taking nine-week old puppy "Murphy" home had arrived. With a big contagious smile on his face he said, "It's so exciting and great because I saw his little face and it just made me smile!" His mother, Kathleen Miller, was happy too. She said, "It is really a difficult time and this has been like a shining moment during that…something you can look forward to." It is not just owning and taking little Murphy home with him that is so meaningful, but Murphy will be his new little friend. "A trip is really nice for memories, but a dog is like years and years with the companionship that they offer" said Storm. "We felt very honored and thrilled to have the opportunity to bring this puppy into our lives," Kathleen stated. This is not just a story about a boy facing cancer; rather it is a story of the hope that God's wisdom brings! *"Eat honey, my son, for it is good; honey from the comb is sweet to your taste. Know also that wisdom is sweet to your soul; if you find it, there is a future hope for you, and your hope will not be cut off"* (Proverbs 24:13-14). The power of God's wisdom can overcome the humongous discouragements of bad news. Wisdom is pleasing, pleasant and tasty like honey. Did you see it in this story?

Here are some examples:

- Changing our focus to what is good brings goodwill. Helping Storm focus on what is good—a puppy—brought goodwill! *"He who seeks good finds goodwill, but evil comes to him who searches for it"* (Proverbs 11:27).

- *"A happy heart makes the face cheerful...A cheerful look brings joy to your heart. And good news gives health to your body"* (Proverbs 15:13, 30). Storm's smile showed his happiness and was a sign he felt better because of little "Murphy." If you saw his smile you would be smiling too!

- The gift of little "Murphy" gives Storm the opportunity to feed, hold and train him. *"Your own soul is nourished when you are kind"* (Proverbs 11:17). *"Being kind to the needy brings happiness"* (Proverbs 14:21). Kindness to needy people, and needy puppies, brings benefits to the giver!

- *"Wisdom is supreme; therefore get wisdom"* (Proverbs 4:7). One reason for its supremacy is how these teachings benefit our own health and well-being. *"Do not let them out of your sight, keep them within your heart; for they are life to those who find them and health to one's whole body"* (Proverbs 4:21-22). Watch Storm's smile at http://wlns. com/2016/06/10/a-teen-a-puppy-and-a-wish-granted/

COPING WITH STORMS

"Severe storms forecasted!" That phrase causes anxiety, precaution, change of plans, and frustration. Right when a meeting started Tuesday evening, I received a phone call about the imminent threat of hail. Cancel the meeting and get out of there was the message! We did. Storms also bring an emotional response of what is really important. One family's house near Luther had its roof ripped off by a tornado. The family had moved into the house just last December. When the owner was interviewed, he relayed that when they realized a tornado was on the way they were able to seek shelter in a neighbor's basement. The peculiar thing about the storm was that it only hit their house. Everyone else was spared in the neighborhood. No bitterness was expressed but instead the memorable phrase was "you can replace things, but not people." He was thankful his family safely made it through the ordeal.

A storm gives a miniature portrait of life. Life involves thinking, planning, preparing and prioritizing. It involves resilience and flexibility. We see all these characteristics taught as "skills for living" in God's wisdom. *"A good person gives life to others; the wise person teaches others how to live"* Proverbs 11:30.

Thinking: *"The wisdom of the prudent is to give **thought** to their ways, but the folly of fools is deception"* Proverbs 14:8.

Planning: *"The **plans** of the diligent lead to profit as surely as haste leads to poverty"* Proverbs 21:5.

Preparing: *"My son, if you **accept** my words and **store up** my commands within you, **turning** your ear to wisdom and **applying** your heart to understanding...Discretion will protect you, and understanding will guard you"* Proverbs 2:1-2,11.

Prioritizing: *"Finish your outdoor work. Get your fields ready. After that, build your house"* Proverbs 24:27.

Resilience: *"For though a righteous man **falls seven times, he rises again,** but the wicked are brought down by calamity"* Proverbs 24:16.

Flexibility: *"The way of fools seems right to them, but the wise listen to advice"* Proverbs 12:15.

We, being trained in the way of wisdom, are to teach wisdom, let people know of dangers and how to live. *"A wise man's heart guides his mouth, and his **lips promote instruction"*** Proverbs 16:23. We can cope with the storms of life, just like literal storms, when we put into practice *"the way of wisdom"* Proverbs 4:11. Jesus says of those who practice his wisdom *"They are like a man building a house, who dug down deep and laid the foundation* *on rock. When a flood came, the torrent struck that house but could not shake it, because it was well built"* Luke 6:46.

CHANGE IS HERE (HEAR)

Change isn't always easy to accomplish. Change may require removing comfortable routines or habits. Change needs to happen when those habits aren't for our well-being. Change can then bring greater health, wellness, progress, and even new horizons and new experiences.

Several examples amplify the wonderful results that change brings. Baby Jordan was born with hearing loss. Giggles bubbled out his mouth when he heard his mother's voice for the first time at three months old. At the age of seven years Myridith clearly heard for the first time. Born moderately deaf she could only hear muffled sounds. When she heard clearly for the first time, joy and happiness radiated from her face. Both of these children experienced clear hearing from the gifts of hearing aids.

Sarah, with severe hearing impairment, received a cochlear implant when she was 29. She said, "Half of me was just scared to death that it was going to come on and I wasn't going to like it, just because...this is all I've ever known for 29 years. So, the fear of the unknown, not knowing what it was going to sound like, can be overwhelming. And it was just nervousness, (but) then the other half of me, 'Oh hurry up and turn it on!'" Her husband video recorded when the implant was turned on. She burst into tears, covering her mouth and then hearing herself talk for the first time. She says "I don't want to hear myself cry," and then broke out in laughter.

Change brought joy to all of them! God's wisdom can reward, strengthen, encourage and bring peace, joy and health too. *"Whoever gives heed to instruction prospers, and blessed is he who trusts in the LORD"* (Proverbs 16:20). *"He who gets wisdom loves his own soul; he who cherishes understanding prospers"* (Proverbs 19:8). The use of "prosper" in these verses includes qualities of health, wellness, happiness and safety.

When we know certain habits are harmful, stop them! *"A prudent man sees danger and takes refuge, but the simple keep going and suffer for it"* (Proverbs 22:3).

When we have the opportunity to help, do so! *"Whenever you are able, do good to people who need help. If you have what your neighbor asks for, don't say, "Come back later. I will give it to you tomorrow"* (Proverbs 3:27-28).

When we want love and trust, plan for what is good! *"...Those who plan to do good will be loved and trusted"* (Proverbs 14:22).

Change is so good when that change is for our well-being!

Watch: "Three-Month-Old Australian Baby Jordan Hears For The First Time" at https://www.youtube.com/watch?v=ImTRWOhzCRw

Watch: "Seven-year-old girl hears clearly" at http://nbc4i.com/2016/07/21/watch-the-moment-7-year-old-girl-gets-gift-of-hearing/

Watch: "29 years old and hearing myself for first time" at https://www.youtube.com/watch?v=LsOo3jzkhYA

INTEGRITY

"Sticks and stones may break my bones, but words will never hurt me" is an old adage we've all heard. Is it true? It wasn't true in the following story of Josh and Leonard. Leonard, who is seventy-five, sits on his front porch most of the day. Josh, who is a thirty-five-year old track inspector, walks past Leonard's house each day on his way to meet other workers of the Union Pacific Railroad. In silence they greet each other with a wave and a smile.

On one day, Josh heard two teenage boys ridicule the looks of Leonard's house by yelling toward him that it should be burned to the ground. Josh saw Leonard's head drop, as those mocking words hurt. Those disrespectful comments affected Josh too.[8]

For a couple of days, he thought about this mistreatment and considered that no elderly person should ever have to endure hearing such words. He remembered he was taught to respect people and help those who don't have much. After mulling over the situation for a couple of days, he decided to do something about the house. To be able to sit on his front porch and feel good about his house is what he wanted for Leonard. Josh called a friend, who manages a local lumber and paint store, to ask for help. He agreed to supply materials. The next day Josh knocked on Leonard's front door, and the silence of four years was finally broken. He asked him if he could paint his house. Leonard excitingly agreed!

Josh needed help; five of his coworkers volunteered. He also posted the situation on his Facebook account. To his surprise, the message was shared more than 6,000 times. On the designated Saturday the six of them showed up to start painting, but to their amazement total strangers also came. Josh stopped counting after ninety-five. The job was done in nine hours. Not only did they repaint the house, but Leonard was given new porch furniture and a new porch for the furniture!

From now on as Josh walks to work he can wave to Leonard, not as a stranger but as a friend. Josh thought what happened was just amazing. He said he had no plan or guidance, but it all came together. However, I see God's wisdom weaved throughout the story. These teachings are either violated or practiced throughout what happened. *"Careless words stab like a sword, but wise words bring healing...It is a sin to belittle one's neighbor; blessed are those who are kind to the needy...What is desirable in a man is his kindness...The integrity of the upright guides them"* Proverbs 12:18, 14:21, 19:22, 11:3. His integrity guided him. He brought healing words of *"*can we paint your house?*"* He didn't belittle his neighbor, but instead honored and respected him. He showed kindness with his offer to paint. Respect, kind words and helpful actions guided him. In other words, his integrity guided him. God's wisdom was woven into his integrity!

WISDOM (THE SKILL FOR LIVING) AND THE PROVERBS
Wisdom was prevalent and relevant in each of the previous stories. They were seen in wisdom sayings or proverbs. Most proverbs are short pithy sayings packed with compressed experience and basic truth that applies to a broad variety of situations. They are wisdom's teachings. The teachings of wisdom empower a person to make changes for resilience, strength and health—the skill for living. *"The teaching of wise people is like a fountain that gives life. It turns those who listen to it away from the*

jaws of death...A good person gives life to others; the wise person teaches others how to live." (Proverbs 13:14 NIrV, 11:30 NCV).

EXPLANATION OF PROVERBS

The word translated "proverb" means "represent," "compare," or be "like." Proverbs in the book of Proverbs give imagery or a picture of reality or life. They are easily repeated and remembered. Here are some examples of pictures they give: *"As a dog returns to its vomit, so fools repeat their folly...As a door turns on its hinges, so a sluggard turns on his bed. A sluggard buries his hand in the dish; he is too lazy to bring it back to his mouth"* (Proverbs 26:11, 14-15).

THE PROVERBS PRESCRIPTIONS
FOR HEALTH AND WELLNESS

"My son, pay attention to what I say; turn your ear to my words. Do not let them out of your sight, keep them within your heart; for they are life to those who find them and health to one's whole body" (Proverbs 4: 20-22). *"A generous person will prosper* (be healthy); *whoever refreshes others will be refreshed"* (Proverbs 11: 25). *"A sluggard's appetite is never filled, but the desires of the diligent* (those who plan ahead) *are fully satisfied* (healthy)" (Proverbs 13: 4). *"Peace of mind means a healthy body, but jealousy will rot your bones"* (Proverbs 14: 30 NCV). *"A cheerful look brings joy to your heart. And good news gives health to your body"* (Proverbs 15: 30 NIrV). *"Pleasant words are like honey. They are sweet to the spirit and bring healing to the body"* (Proverbs 16: 24 NIrV). *"The greedy stir up conflict, but those who trust* (have confidence, security) *in the LORD will prosper* (be healthy)" (Proverbs 28: 25).

INTERNAL HEALTH DIALOGUE PRESCRIPTION FOR PEOPLE WITH DIABETES

As a man steps off the curb and begins to walk across the street, a car comes screeching around the corner. The car is coming straight toward the man. He picks up his pace, trying to hurry across the street. The car changes lanes and comes straight toward him. So, he turns around to go back, but the car changes lanes too. The car is so close and the man is so scared that he just freezes in his tracks. The car swerves at the last moment just missing the man and screeches to a stop. The window comes down. The driver is a squirrel and says, "See, it's not as easy as it looks, is it?"

Maybe there was a time when you thought someone ought to be handling some stressful situation better. After experiencing something similar, you found out that "it's not as easy as it looks." Without actually experiencing something there is no way to understand what it exactly feels like.

When I look at people who struggle with their diabetes to control their blood sugars, I know from my own experience that "it's not as easy as it looks." So, I want to make it easier with tips and ideas from my own experience as well as research. We need motivation to do the right things which we can build with God's wisdom! As you continue to read this book, you will notice how God's wisdom intricately applies to life's situations and how that wisdom directly relates to our health. What I experience each day illustrates how the Proverbs and wisdom apply.

When I get up in the morning the first thing on my mind is blood sugar. What is my blood glucose level? Is it high, low or is it just right? So, I check my blood glucose first thing in the morning. Then throughout the day those thoughts stay with me. After eating lunch, I wonder if I took enough insulin for the carbohydrates I ate. If I'm not wearing my continuous glucose monitor sensor, I'm checking what my blood sugar is. So, I check myself multiple times a day, think about the amount of exercise I'm getting and the amount of carbohydrates I'm eating.

I do this to make sure I'm getting the proper balance of food, activity and insulin to maintain blood sugar levels as close to normal as possible. Do I succeed? Not always. You may think—what an annoyance, nuisance or hassle! Is that anyway to live a life? Yes, because to think this way is the "way of wisdom." Proverbs 4:23 states *"Be careful what you think, because your thoughts run your life."* These are pleasant words or thoughts and God's wisdom states *"Pleasant words are like honey. They are sweet to the spirit and bring healing to the body"* (Proverbs 16:24).

This doesn't mean throughout the day I'm thinking of nothing else. If you are not thinking about your health though, what you are eating, how many steps you're taking, then start. It is the "way of wisdom." And as I've mentioned, wisdom is "the skill for living."

> *"Keep their words in mind forever as though you had them tied around your neck. They will guide you when you walk. They will guard you when you sleep. They will speak to you when you are awake"* (Proverbs 6:21-22).

CHAPTER ONE

The Power of Optimism

---

*The spirit of a man will sustain him in sickness, But
who can bear a broken spirit?* (Proverbs 18:14 NKJV)

When it comes to blood sugar control for diabetes I've seen
and heard people in frustration just openly give up. "I
never check myself. It is too expensive and I'm always high
anyway." Or "I'm always in such pain and nothing I do seems
to make any difference." Or "I do everything right. I check my
blood sugar and it is 120. I eat nothing and less than two hours
later I'm 269. This is so discouraging why even try?" With a
frustrated, discouraged attitude many people I've known in the
almost six decades I've had diabetes have just given up. I know it
can be frustrating because the 120 to 269 blood glucose example
is mine, but I'm not giving up!

People with diabetes express their frustration with all the
things they should do—checking blood glucose levels, following a meal plan that involves avoiding certain foods, counting

carbohydrates, taking medications or insulin and moving more! One person came to a diabetes support group meeting hoping to get some help. She lashed out at what she had to do. She was cussing at the diabetes for what it was doing to her, not realizing she could outsmart diabetes. She came to a few meetings and then stopped coming, not wanting to be around people who were facing some of the complications and challenges she was facing. She didn't want to be reminded of what she had! She just gave up and died of complications three years later. Most people who come to a diabetes support group are there to learn and be encouraged. We like encouragement; we like to hear about people who overcome hardships. The way of wisdom teaches how important words are. *"Anxiety weighs down the heart, but a kind word cheers it up"* (Proverbs 12:25). We need to hear words that boost and promote a positive attitude, words that lift us up! Words reflect how we think, what our attitude is. Consider the following poem "The man who thinks he can" by Walter D. Wintle.

THE MAN WHO THINKS HE CAN

If you think you are beaten, you are; If you think you dare not, you don't. If you'd like to win, but you think you can't, It is almost a cinch that you won't.

If you think you'll lose, you're lost; For out of the world we find. Success begins with a fellow's will; It's all in the state of mind.

If you think you're outclassed, you are; You've got to think high to rise. You've got to be sure of yourself before You can ever win the prize.

Life's battles don't always go to the stronger and faster man, But sooner or later the man who wins Is the man who thinks he can.

What is said in that poem is similar to God's wisdom, which teaches, *"Be careful what you think, because your thoughts run your life"* (Proverbs 4:23).

Does attitude make a difference when confronted with a disease? The way of wisdom answers back with a resounding yes! Yes, it makes a difference! *"The spirit of a man will sustain him in sickness, but who can bear a broken spirit?"* Or *"The will to live can get you through sickness, but no one can live with a broken spirit"* (Proverbs 18:14 NKJV, NCV).

ARE WE GOING TO JUST SIT DOWN AND GIVE UP OR STAND UP AND FIGHT?

Is it better to just sit passively and accept whatever illness or disease is diagnosed? Or is it better to do all we can to outsmart the disease? In other words, are we going to just sit down and give up or stand up and fight? I've been striving to outsmart diabetes now for almost six decades. What that means is that I've had to fight diabetes by checking my blood glucose more than 100,000 times, take more than 43,000 injections (would have been more if I hadn't used an insulin pump for the last fifteen years), follow a meal plan, stay on the move every day and cope with some diabetes complications. A book that intrigued me years ago about this concept of attitude and involvement was "Anatomy of an Illness" by Norman Cousins.

Norman Cousins was diagnosed with an excruciating painful illness with a high sedimentation rate that indicated inflammatory activity in his body. He wasn't going to just sit in a hospital passively lying there though. Instead he bolstered a positive attitude in a number of ways. His condition was diagnosed as "a serious collagen illness-a disease of the connective tissue." [9] Experts gave him one chance in 500 for recovery.

Fight the diagnosed disease is what he did by reinforcing a positive attitude. He wrote, "The inevitable question arose in my mind: what about the positive emotions? If negative emotions produce negative chemical changes in the body, wouldn't the positive emotions produce positive chemical changes? Is it possible that love, hope, faith, laughter, confidence, and the will to live have therapeutic value?" [10] One of the ways he discovered to alleviate pain was through laughter. He also had a doctor, William Hitzig, who was a partner, not a dictator in facing his illness.

Doctor Charles Fletcher, a chest physician expressed the importance of working with patients instead of just dictating in 1982. He himself has had diabetes for forty years when he wrote this.

"We doctors who have to manage chronic disabling conditions should pay far more attention to the importance to patients of their being independent of as many restrictions as possible, and we should encourage them to be original in their self-management. We should more often ask the question 'How do you feel about your illness?' or 'What bothers you most about your treatment?'" [11]

Mr. Cousins drew several conclusions about his illness and treatment. His will to live and his involvement in the methods of treatment were therapeutic. Some doctors commented that he was a "beneficiary of a mammoth venture in self-administered placebos." He said, "Such a hypothesis bothers me not at all."[12] He knew that attitude can make a difference! Several years after writing his book he became a senior lecturer for ten years at the UCLA School of Medicine. He interviewed hundreds of patients, medical doctors and students and research scientists. Here is a typical example of one of those interviews that reveals the importance of attitude.

The interview was with the father and his twenty-six-year old son who was diagnosed with MS. He had pains that had come and gone for half a year. He was then sent to a specialist, a neurologist. "It all happened so quickly," he said. "One day I was in charge of my life. I was confident that my pains would lesson. Then the next day I was terribly sick, hardly able to move. My pains were awful, especially in my legs and my back." His father had accompanied him. When he was diagnosed he saw changes in his son immediately. After the diagnosis he seemed to age by twenty years. He walked out of the office like an old man. Agony was in every step. The next morning, he couldn't get up. He seemed paralyzed.

When the diagnosis was given his attitude changed. He walked into the office seeming to do ok. Then when the diagnosis was given he could barely walk. Hope is what he really wanted in looking at his newly diagnosed illness. So, Cousins arranged for him to meet a physician who was extraordinarily compassionate with good communication skills. He had a way of reassuring people! Cousins also arranged for him to meet with several survivors with the same condition to help enhance his attitude and comply with medical treatment.[13]

We all need hope! God and his wisdom give us hope. *"Eat honey, my son, for it is good; honey from the comb is sweet to your taste. Know also that wisdom is like honey for you: If you find it, there is a future hope for you, and your hope will not be cut off"* (Proverbs 24:13-14). Compassion is God's wisdom. Getting support from others is God's wisdom. The following fundamental way of wisdom instructions relate to hope, support and wellbeing. *"Do not forget my teaching, but keep my commands in your heart, for they will prolong your life many years and bring you peace and prosperity...Whenever you are able, do good to people who need help...Anxiety weighs down the heart, but a kind word cheers it up...It is a sin to despise one's neighbor, but blessed is the one who is kind to the needy"* (Proverbs 3:1-2, 3:27 NCV, 12:25, 14:21).

Notice how wisdom and a positive attitude relates to a teenager who makes a dramatic comeback after a brain injury, a man who is diagnosed with impending blindness when he is in his early twenties, a blind pole vaulter who earns a bronze medal, the glad attitude of a woman celebrating her 104th birthday, and the cheerfulness of a young man working at his restaurant with Down syndrome.

GIVE THOUGHT TO YOUR WAYS: A TEENAGE PITCHER'S COMEBACK

They drive; they run; they get caught. The sequence is repeated over and over again by people who think they can out speed the police. They think if they reach speeds of more than a 100 mph, or even up to 135 mph, they won't get caught. Police chases in Oklahoma City, Tulsa and an even more bizarre case in Los Angeles have captured the news lately. In L.A. instead of trying to run from their car to prevent getting caught they just got out and started taking "selfies" with their phones before and while being arrested. What do they all have in common? Foolishness! *"A prudent man sees danger and takes refuge, but the simple keep going and suffer for it"* Proverbs 22:3.

A large crowd gathered around a 100-foot diving tower at the state fair, waiting for the star performer. Finally, a feeble ninety-nine-year old man walked with his cane to the microphone. He said, "I'm ninety-nine years old and I'm going to amaze you. I'll climb to the top of that tower and dive into this teeny, tiny tub of water. Are you ready to see this outstanding feat?" Everyone gasped and begged him to not do it. He said, "OK, the next performance is at 10 o'clock." It didn't take much to persuade him. We can at least give him credit for giving thought to his ways. *"A simple man believes anything, but a prudent man gives thought to his steps"* Proverbs 14:15.

Another person who really gave thought to his steps was in the news lately. His name is Lance Cotter. His story is impressive and uplifting! This Putnam City pitcher is excelling to major league team considerations. Excel names his attitude because last summer as Lance played catcher a batter swung and hit his head. The hit caused a traumatic brain injury. He was in ICU for seven days suffering from seizures and a stroke. He was determined to not let this tragedy end his career. He has trained and trained for seven months, making a comeback. His coach is impressed with his persistence and work ethic. It is paying off because he thinks the "sky is the limit" for him—he can go as far as he wants to go he feels!

Just like the other examples we've noticed, it comes down to each person's choice. We've seen that thoughtful choices, not foolish impulsive choices, make the best choices! Giving thought to our choices should be the guiding principle for the decisions we make. After all it is written in God's wisdom, *"An upright man gives thought to his ways"* (Proverbs 21:29).

"For through wisdom your days will be many, and years will be added to your life. If you are wise, your wisdom will reward you" (Proverbs 9:11-12).

WHAT WE ARE—OR—WHAT WE HAVE

Thomas A. Edison said, "Your worth consists in what you are and not in what you have." Are we kind, generous, patient, thankful, humble, considerate, self-controlled, forgiving, honest, persevering and reliable? Do we have a large house, a nice car and a big bank account? The answer to those two questions is the difference of being or having and will determine how we cope. A person can have an abundance of material things and not be generous, thankful and considerate. Many are devastated when storms destroy the things they have, their homes, cars and other possessions.

Are we discerning like one man after a hurricane destroyed everything he had? In an interview he said, "We have lost just about everything." However, he chuckled and looked at his family and said, "But I guess we got out with about everything that matters." He was wise and realized what really matters.

What people are makes the difference on how they cope with loss. In 1976, one young man named Jim Stovall was diagnosed with a rare eye disease. It was discovered during a routine check-up before he entered college, and eventually led to his blindness. As a teenager with his entire life ahead of him it was what he called an "indescribable devastation." How did he cope with the difficult loss of his eyesight? Did he give up on life? The answer is a resounding "No!" He went on to become a national champion Olympic weightlifter, an Emmy Award winner, the president of a television network, one of the Ten Outstanding Young Americans, and the national Entrepreneur of the Year. But more important than those personal achievements, is his encouragement to others as an author.

One of the books he authored was "The Ultimate Gift" which was made into an outstanding movie that I highly recommend. It was about a young man who was to inherit a great fortune from his grandfather if he realized the importance of being rather than having. Certain tests about his quality of character and attitude toward life were to be passed before he could receive his inheritance. These were termed "gifts" like the gift of gratitude, work, learning, giving, love and even problems.

As we look for God's wisdom, we see this concept in what Paul wrote to the church at Corinth two thousand years ago. He doesn't write about the value of things, but about the value of the attributes of love. *"Love is patient, love is kind. It does not envy, it does not boast, it is not proud. It is not rude, it is not self-seeking, it is not easily angered, it keeps no record of wrongs. Love does not delight in evil but rejoices with the truth. It always protects, always trusts, always hopes, always perseveres. Love never fails"* (1 Corinthians 13:4-7). Yes, Mr. Edison had insight when he said, "Your worth consists in what you are and not in what you have."

> **Watch:** "The Ultimate Gift—Official Movie Trailer" https://www.youtube.com/watch?v=rwXe5eKZr6M and "Jim Stovall—Christopher Story" https://www.youtube.com/watch?v=q1xGJZngN5g

WISDOM, HEALTH AND WELLNESS APPLICATION

A study was done at Cal-Davis University by Dr. Emmons on perceiving good things as gifts. Half of the gifts listed related to "interpersonal" or "spiritual" categories. When these categories were viewed not as just good things, but as gifts, the participants were able to come up with 20 percent more things to list. According to the research, these are the categories of blessings that relate to better health and well-being. Research also indicated that the more a receiver valued the gift, the greater he or she experienced gratitude. Instead of just thinking of oral medications, glucose meters and checking strips, insulin, knowledge of the glycemic index—in other words, the resources that were not even available years ago for people to use—as merely good things, think of them as gifts. And let's not forget to cherish the supportive people in our lives as gifts as well!

BLIND POLE VAULTER WINS STATE CHAMPIONSHIP'S BRONZE

A headline reads "Blind pole vaulter Charlotte Brown wins state championships bronze." This happened in Texas recently when

Charlotte Brown vaulted 11'6" to win third place in the finals and she is legally blind. "This story really wasn't about me," said the 17-year-old. "It was about everybody that struggles with something." The Emory Rains student has pursued a medal for the past two years, finishing eighth and then fourth before taking third as a high school senior. Brown first took up pole vaulting, which is now a Paralympic sport, in seventh grade.

How can a blind person pole vault you may wonder? She counts the seven steps of her left foot on her approach. She then listens for the sound of a faint beeper placed on the mat that tells her when to plant the pole and push up. "It took me three years to get on the podium, and I finally did it," she said. "If I could send a message to anybody, it's not about pole vaulting and it's not about track. It's about finding something that makes you happy despite whatever obstacles are in your way."

What can make us happy is to serve the Lord using the guidance and encouragement he gives us through his word. Yes, we face obstacles that get in the way, but God's word says *"Let us not become weary in doing good, for at the proper time **we will reap a harvest if we do not give up"** (Galatians 6:9).

P.S.: You can watch her vault at: https://www.youtube.com/watch?v=YQaHKbJjhuw

WOMAN CELEBRATES HER 104th BIRTHDAY WITH GLADNESS

I was reading about a Fort Worth woman who was celebrating her 104th year of life. "Well at 103 I didn't think I'd make it, but I'm still perking along," she said. At 104 years old, Elizabeth

Sullivan says she doesn't need the advice of real doctors. Instead she keeps another kind of doctor near. "People try to give me coffee for breakfast. Well, I'd rather have a Dr. Pepper." She said, "I started drinking them about 40 years ago, three a day. Every doctor that sees me says they'll kill you, but they die and I don't. So, there must be a mistake somewhere."

For her birthday on March 18th she got a beautiful cake shaped like the can of a Dr. Pepper. Commenting on her birthday celebration she said, "When you live to be 104 and still can talk to nice people, you deserve some Dr. Pepper, but I never expected this. I'm feeling good. I'm glad I'm still here. I'm glad I'm not in a rest home. Glad I can read books and watch TV and have people come by and say hello." When she was asked if she had a secret for living past 100, she said that she really didn't except "You just keep living." However, after watching and listening to what she had to say I see her enjoyment of life and attitude of gratitude extending her life. You can view the interview at **https://www.youtube.com/watch?v=vBwSeITMmJA**. Shouldn't we too be grateful and glad?

Paul writes, *"Rejoice in the Lord always. I will say it again: Rejoice!"* (Philippians 4:4) God's wisdom also tells us that being glad is good medicine. *"A glad heart makes a healthy body, but a crushed spirit makes the bones dry"* or *"A merry heart does good, like medicine, but a broken spirit dries the bones"* (Proverbs 17:22 NKJV). Of course, one of the ways we can be glad is to focus on the good things that happen to us each day and be thankful. Wasn't that the attitude of Elizabeth Sullivan on her 104th birthday? Let's make that our attitude each day as well!

> *"A cheerful look brings joy to your heart. And good news gives health to your body"* (Proverbs 15:30).

A CHEERFUL HEART IS GOOD MEDICINE

"A cheerful heart is good medicine, but a crushed spirit dries up the bones" (Proverbs 17:22). We all like to be healthy and that verse tells us how—with a cheerful heart. A cheerful attitude strengthens our mental, emotional and physical lives with optimism. A cheerful attitude overcomes a crushed, discouraged attitude. How is a cheerful heart possible? Do circumstances have to fit perfectly together to have a cheerful heart? *"Those who plan what is good find love and faithfulness"* (Proverbs 14:22). Planning and doing are found in this good medicine.

Breakfast is my favorite meal of the day. Many restaurants have a variety of delicious food they offer, but have you ever seen a menu that comes with hugs. Hugs? Yes, hugs. Hugs are on the menu at Tim's Place, a restaurant in Albuquerque, New Mexico. Tim is the owner and, although he has Down syndrome, he was able to go to college and graduated in 2008. He majored in food service, office skills and restaurant hosting.

His family helped him start the restaurant in 2010. For over ten years he dreamed of owning his own business and now he does. He claims his restaurant is the world's friendliest. What makes it the friendliest has to do with his favorite part of his work day—giving out his "Tim hugs" for free. After being in business for three years he had given 40,000 hugs. A digital display on the wall shows the number of hugs, and after five years he had given out 75,402 hugs.

Family Therapist, Virginia Satir, says "We need 4 hugs a day for survival. We need 8 hugs a day for maintenance. We need 12 hugs a day for growth." Dr. Rock of the Cleveland Clinic says that hugs can decrease release of cortisol (a stress hormone), lower blood pressure, slow heart rate in stressful situations, and strengthen the immune system. With Tim's favorite time at work he was promoting health in his customers. No wonder they loved him.

How can we have the good medicine of a cheerful heart? Let's follow Tim's example of cheer and thankfulness. He loved his job and customers; he gave cheer to others with his hugs. *"A cheerful look brings joy to your heart. And good news gives health to your body"* (Proverbs 15:30 NIrV). Tim was making good news with his hugs. After five years he closed the doors of his restaurant. Why? He wanted to marry someone he loved more—his girlfriend, Tiffani Johnson. They met at a Down syndrome convention. He's married now living in Denver and hopes to open another restaurant there.

Watch an interview with Tim at "Historic roadside restaurant plans to stop taking orders" https://www.youtube.com/watch?v=K_zKjNqmMjl and https://www.youtube.com/watch?v=ttZPj2XwVH8

EMOTIONAL BURDEN OF CHRONIC DISEASES

When I looked at the people in the previous examples, I was encouraged and I hope you were too! We all need encouragement. If they can face their challenges with a positive attitude so can we. Emotional burdens come with chronic diseases like diabetes. I'm not saying that just from my own experience but from research of thousands of people.

HEALTH APPLICATIONS TO BUILD A POSITIVE ATTITUDE

The study "Diabetes Attitudes, Wishes and Needs" was conducted in 2011 with almost 8600 people with both Type 1 and Type 2 Diabetes. The study was done primarily in North America and Europe. The study revealed attitudes that need to be strengthened as well as coping with challenging needs.

People answered open-ended questions about impacting experiences, challenges they faced, successes and wishes for personal improvement. Such things as not always having to be on guard, the wish for less anxiety and worry were expressed. Fifty-six percent were afraid and one of the big fears was hypoglycemia. One elderly woman expressed this fear by saying, "I was living by myself and I had a hypoglycemic crisis. I was no longer able to understand anything; they told me I did not make sense when I talked and that I wasn't able to move, to sleep calmly, to recognize my children."[14] (Read how I treat hypoglycemia in chapter nine, number 16 of wise ways to outsmart diabetes.) Forty-five per cent hoped for "less anxiety and worry," as in "I wish I didn't have to have my guard up." One woman said, "This illness makes me very afraid, even if I am used to it." Others were afraid they would not be able to control their diabetes.

What caught my attention too were the negative moods of people—even a sense of hopelessness. One person said, "When everything is going well, I am well and so is the diabetes. On the other hand, however, whenever I have a bout of the blues, or my morale is low, it goes out of whack and the diabetes is like a yo-yo."[15] Is any of this surprising? No, just think of the challenge we all face no matter if it is health issues or other difficult situations. We need a positive attitude and the following three ways will help build that attitude—gratitude, humor and singing.

"The spirit of a man will sustain him in sickness, but who can bear a broken spirit?" (Proverbs 18:14 NKJV).

THE GRATITUDE PRESCRIPTION

Why be thankful? It has been said that our minds are like Velcro for negative information but like Teflon for positive. You've probably noticed how easy it is to focus on the negative. The difference between a positive or a pessimistic attitude can come from where we focus. Consider this story. Years ago, a woman lived in a one-room shack with her husband and children. It was so crowded; she didn't know how much longer she could stand it. An old sage lived nearby with a reputation for giving valuable advice. She went to him, told him of her situation, and asked what she could do.

"Do you have any chickens," he asked. She said, "Yes." "Bring those chickens into the house and come back in one week." When she came back, she told him it was horrible. She thought her situation was now unbearable! Even though he heard her answer, he asked "Do you own a cow." She said, "Yes." "Bring that cow into the house also for the next week and then come back." She reluctantly did so with grave doubts and sure enough her situation only got worse. She came back admitting,

"I'm at my wits end. I can't stand it any longer." The sage wasn't surprised. In fact, that is just what he expected. He told her to remove the chickens and the cow then to come again in a week. This time he was confronted with a beaming, radiant face! She couldn't hide how ecstatic she was with her one-room shack! Nothing had changed. The room was the same size. Only her attitude had changed. When she realized what she really had, it was good news and she was so thankful. Let's focus on good news too! That is the point of gratitude—to realize what we have. When we do, research indicates our health and well-being will improve. The way of wisdom teaches this too. *"A cheerful look brings joy to your heart. And good news gives health to your body"* (Proverbs 15:30 NIrV).

Count your blessing, name them one by one will make a difference in your health according to research done by professor Robert Emmons of the University of California at Davis. In his ten-week research study hundreds of participants demonstrated that counting good things does make a difference. They were randomly divided into three groups—gratitude, hassle and neutral groups. The gratitude condition group was to list five things for which they could be thankful that had affected their lives from the previous week. The hassle group was to do the same thing but with five burdens that affected their lives the previous week. The third group, the neutral group was also to list five things but in their case the things could be positive or negative.

The results were then analyzed with several tests. The final analysis was that the people in the gratitude group felt better about their lives, were more optimistic, and exercised more than those in the other groups.[16]

A similar ten-week study by the Department of Physical Medicine and Rehabilitation at the University involved people with post-polio syndrome. The gratitude group results were feeling better about themselves, more optimistic about the coming week, and more connected with others than the other groups. They were also able to get to sleep quicker, spent more time sleeping, and felt more refreshed in the morning.[17] To sleep more soundly one should count blessings instead of sheep.

Research indicates several health benefits for being grateful. Emotional well-being, getting along better with others, more resilient to trauma, less depressed, more generous and helpful to others and less likely to burn out are just some of the benefits. Obviously, counting blessings sounds better than meditating on problems.

What should we count when it comes to blessings—little and insignificant things? Taking them for granted is easy, but instead focusing on the trivial helps! Count them. List them. Pray about them each day—before going to bed or when getting up. A potentially "gloomy day" will turn "into a bright shiny day!" A good day will result when we do a variety of things using our hands, seeing the beauty of flowers, enjoying the aroma and taste of delicious food and doing it all with gratitude! To see, walk, taste, feel, "eat, as well as have a home," bed, clothes, family and friends are the little things that we can appreciate, count and list for a good day! Pleasant thinking and words is what this is.

"Pleasant words are like honey. They are sweet to the spirit and bring healing to the body" (Proverbs 16:24 NIrV).

THE HUMOR PRESCRIPTION

"Warning: Humor may be hazardous to your illness."

In his 1928 book "Laughter and Health" Dr. James J. Walsh wrote, "The mental effect (of laughter) brushes away the dreads and fears which constitute the basis of so many diseases and complaints, and lifts men out of the slough of despond into which they are so likely to fall when they take themselves too seriously."

Almost 3,000 years ago, which is long before 1928, Solomon wrote about cheerfulness. *"A cheerful heart is good medicine, but a crushed spirit dries up the bones"* (Proverbs 17:22). *"A happy heart makes the face cheerful, but heartache crushes the spirit...All the days of the oppressed are wretched, but the cheerful heart has a continual feast"* (Proverbs 15:13,15). *"A cheerful look brings joy to your heart. And good news gives health to your body"* (Proverbs 15:30 NIrV).

A sense of humor, a positive attitude, support of friends and laughter itself can bring health benefits. In 1988 Dr. Marvin E. Herring, at New Jersey's School of Osteopathic Medicine, explains "The diaphragm, thorax, abdomen, heart, lungs and even the liver are given a massage during a hearty laugh."[18]

Norman Cousins used laughter like a medicine for fighting his painful illness. Part of his diet was viewing comedies. He watched Marx Brothers films and episodes of Candid Camera. By doing this he felt better and discovered about ten minutes of laughter gave him two hours of pain-free sleep. Listen to a boring lecture or watch a comedy, which sounds more appealing to you? Nineteen people with diabetes listened to a boring lecture one day and watched a comedy the next day. They ate the exact same food and amounts each day. Their blood glucose levels were lower after viewing the comedy compared to after listening to a boring lecture![19]

Is humor a character strength? Yes, research indicates that people with a good sense of humor focus on pleasant aspects of life. Thus, it helps a person build friendships, feel better and cope with stress.[20] Even a smile has health benefits. A research study called "Grin and Bear It" revealed that a smile can have a positive cardiovascular influence on the stress response. After doing two stressful tasks heart rates were lower in the smile groups. Chopsticks placed in mouths formed a facial smile. The same was done for another group, but they were also told to smile. Their smile was more of a "Duchenne Smile" where more facial muscles are used. It proved to be the most effective with lower heart rates after the stressful tasks. Smiling and even consciously forming a smile was a stress relief.[21]

JOKES BRING SMILES AND LAUGHTER

One guy liked to use his smart phone and show pictures on it. He asked a friend if he had seen the pictures of his grandchildren. He said he hadn't and he appreciated it! Ha,Ha.

A man was walking in a park. He saw a man sitting on a bench and admired the dog sitting next to the bench. He asked him if his dog bites and he said no. But when he reached down to pet the dog it nearly bit his hand off. "I thought you said your dog doesn't bite!" The man looking down at the dog said, "That ain't my dog!" Amusing things can happen in parks and restaurants. In fact, they can happen about anywhere, if we are looking for them.

My dad has always had a sense of humor. His motto is "we all need humor." He usually has something amusing to say. When we celebrated his 87th birthday, he said, "This is the best 87th birthday I've ever had!" While sitting at a restaurant and being thankful for good lighting at that table, my dad told the following story: One guy as he was travelling saw some horses for sale. He had been searching for another horse so he stopped and inquired what horses were available. He decided on a certain horse and asked the owner about him. The owner couldn't understand why he wanted that one and replied, "He doesn't look very well." The guy purchased him anyway, but the very next day came back. He angrily said, "You sold me a blind horse and didn't tell me." "I did too! I told you he doesn't look very well."

While waiting on the bill and considering the tip for the wait-ress, this story came to his mind. A travelling preacher went to a congregation. It was suggested that a contribution be taken for the preaching and the preacher could just pass his hat. So, the hat was passed through the crowd. After it was returned to him he offered a prayer. When he looked in the hat and found noth-ing, he prayed "Thank you, Lord, that I at least got my hat back."

While eating at another restaurant, we heard: One preacher decided he needed to retire. Why are you going to retire? For health concerns! The church is sick of me…and I'm sick of them! One young farmer looked into the clouds and saw the clouds in the shape of two letters GP. He pondered what that could mean and said to an older farmer "I think it must mean Go Preach" but the farmer thought it probably meant Go Plow.

He would always have fun teasing waiters and waitresses with his sons at restaurants. One time the waiter asked them if they were father and son. And dad who was 86 said he was the son and his son Max who was 65 was his father. This was on a Father's Day. The waiter may have believed him because when they were about to leave he leaned down to look at Max face-to-face and said sincerely, "Have a good Father's Day!"

People were asking dad how he was doing. "I got shot last week, but I think I'll be ok." Everyone showed grave concern and would seriously ask, "You got shot! What happened?" "My leg was in such pain, I got an orthopedic painkiller shot to get some relief." His son recently came down with a cold and was taking medication. He told him that by taking medication a cold will only last a week, but without medication it will last seven days! Dad went to an orthopedic surgeon because of pain in his hip. He dreaded surgery, but after several x-rays the need for surgery was ruled out. He was elated. The doctor prescribed some ointment for him to use on his hip. He then told me that he had heard the cure for the Swine Flu was oinkment!

He told the story about dogs: Two dog owners met in the park one day and each commented on what a beautiful dog the other had. Questions arose on what they fed their dogs. One owner said he only fed his beautiful dog the best dog food that money can buy, but that he's about to eat him out of house and home. The other owner said he fed his dog "turnip greens." "Turnip greens, my beautiful dog would never eat turnip greens." The other owner said, "Mine wouldn't either, the first two weeks."

Dad even sees benefits for being a senior citizen. Some of those benefits are silver in your hair, gold in your mouth, and a senior discount at the golden arches! Another joke he told regarding old age was a conversation two-men were having about underwear, yes underwear. One man asked, "Do you use briefs or boxer shorts?" "Depends!" Yes, my dad says "we all need humor" and we can read such a prescription in God's wisdom. *"A cheerful heart is good medicine, but a crushed spirit dries up the bones"* (Proverbs 17:22). For some really good laughs watch the following two videos:

- "Jim Gaffigan—Bacon—KING BABY" https://www.youtube.com/watch?v=CaK9bjLy3v4

- "Jim Stovall-Blind Guy Meets Deaf Guy Story" https://www.youtube.com/watch?v=_MaguhFCQko

THE SINGING PRESCRIPTION

Research indicates that singing can have positive effects on a person's health. When nursing-home residents participated in a month long singing program levels of anxiety and depression were decreased.[22] Stacy Horn wrote, "What researchers are beginning to discover is that singing is like an infusion of the perfect tranquilizer, the kind that both soothes your nerves and elevates your spirits."[23] Singing can be an anti-depressant because it stimulates the body to release endorphins, the body's natural pain relievers which can also cause feelings of happiness.[24]

I saw the difference singing can make first hand with my father-in-law. His health was declining rapidly in his last few weeks while living at an assisted living facility. One day while his wife of sixty-four years was there visiting she sang "Victory in

Jesus" to him. He knew each word and would form them on his lips as he sang in bed. The next day my wife and I sang that same song to him. He had refused to eat lunch that day; he was lying lethargic in his bed. As we began to sing "Victory in Jesus," he started forming the words on his lips and he was revived. The nurses put him in his recliner and he was ready to eat! From that day on we sang to him every time we went to see him. His three grandsons joined us one Saturday to sing five songs to him. I asked him after each song if he knew it. He said "yep, sort of" and then after we sang "Jesus Loves Me" he said "Of Course!" Those were the only words he could say, he was so weak. I saw how he was revived after these singing sessions and how God's wisdom was coming true. Proverbs 16:24 says, *"Pleasant words are like honey. They are sweet to the spirit and bring healing to the body."* We sang pleasant words to him. So, let's sing and sing to each other.

SING TO EACH OTHER

"Amazing Grace" and "Jesus Loves Me" are often sung within church buildings, but could they also be sung in hospitals? Of course, some nurses sing them to patients to comfort, calm and encourage them. I've discovered that "Singing Nurses" are found in hospitals. Even in a local hospital "Amazing Grace" was sung to calm the patient into compliance to take the medication.

Jared Axen, a registered nurse, likes to sing and purposely uses songs to both relate to and soothe patients. He, at first, would just sing in the hallways until patients started making requests that he start singing to them. Most of his patients have serious health issues and come from 1930s or 1940s. So, he has learned songs from that time period as well as hymns.

He has found that singing is very comforting to his patients. He explained, "When patients are in pain, it gives them some distraction. They may not necessarily be happy about their situation but it seems a little easier [for them] to handle, a little easier to manage." He has found that many need less pain medication as a result of singing.

Each day is important, no matter if you are at the dawn of life or sunset. One nurse wrote, "It is about making those final months, weeks, days, and hours the most meaningful." Singing helps do that. Nurses and staff may sing "Amazing Grace" because a patient requests it. That singing makes a real impact on those in the patient's room and causes a son to comment, "It was beautiful. Mother was weak, but she sang with them." One nurse says, "It's very comforting for [the patients] and you can tell it really brightens their day."

"A cheerful heart is good medicine, but a crushed spirit dries up the bones" (Proverbs 17.22). Singing is one way to make the heart cheerful. Denis Waitley has some good advice. He wrote, "Sing in your car on the way to work. (You may get a few weird stares but only from sour grumps. Others will actually smile and may begin to sing themselves!)...Sing at the top of your lungs. You'll be amazed at how your attitude changes the longer you keep the melody flowing! You'll come away energized."

"Sing psalms, hymns and spiritual songs to each other; sing to the Lord and make music in your heart to him" (Ephesians 5:19).

Watch: Nurse sings "Amazing Grace / My Chains Are Gone" to patient with metastatic lung cancer https://www.youtube.com/watch?v=SXzdMTbpnPl&t=97s

Watch: "Nurse Sings Jesus Loves Me to her Patient" https://www.youtube.com/watch?v=sKWcapbBKwY

Watch: "The Singing Nurse at Valencia hospital soothes the suffering" https://www.youtube.com/watch?v=ODok6eNtA9c&t=11s

Watch: "Nurse uses healing power of song to spread cheer to patients" https://www.youtube.com/watch?v=NXm4SfjW2Bc

CHAPTER TWO

The Power of Kindness

"Your own soul is nourished when you are kind...A generous person will prosper; whoever refreshes others will be refreshed" (Proverbs 11:17,25).

Rescue, observe, care, safety, frantic are all words that fit an alarming event in the news. Travelling at night on an Oregon highway a deputy saw an unbelievable sight. He thought at first it was some sort of animal running down the middle of the highway. His dashboard camera was recording it all as he got closer. He was stunned to see a two-year-old boy running down the highway. The toddler was in danger. The deputy slammed on his breaks. He immediately got out of his car and scooped up the boy as a semi-truck passed nearby.

If the deputy had been distracted and not carefully observing the road that night a tragic story could have unfolded. That little boy, however, was rescued and brought to safety. The deputy soon discovered that his parents were frantically looking for him. He had slipped out of a nearby community center while his parents were cleaning.[25] Watch "Toddler found running down busy highway is saved by police officer" at https://www.youtube.com/watch?v=sni8_4BhqRk

That little boy is like so many people running down the highway of life. They need help! What would you do if you saw a toddler walking on the road? Without hesitation you would stop and rescue him! The Lord tells us that *"what is desirable in a man is his kindness"* (Proverbs 19:22 NASB). Desiring kindness from others is what we all want. Kindness is appreciated. Kindness toward a lost toddler should be easy. Transferring that attitude toward others is needed.

A gem found in God's wisdom is this: *"A **generous** person will **prosper;** whoever refreshes others will be refreshed"* (Proverbs 11:25). The Hebrew word that is translated "prosper" means "to be fat, grow fat, become fat, become prosperous." In other words, in contrast to skin and bones "prosper" is healthy, not wealthy!

We've all found times when we need refreshment in life! Have you ever been in a hospital bed, asking for help and no one comes? Anguish is easy in situations where you are seemingly ignored. I've been there! I read about a surgeon who became the patient. The doctor was recovering from surgery, immobile and in need of a helping hand. He surprisingly received it at the start of the 6:30 morning shift. In walks a nurse making her morning rounds, checking on him. She is about to leave, but then she suddenly stops! She goes over to the sink and moistens a clean washcloth with warm water. She then goes over to him and wipes his face and her only words to him are "This must be hard for you." In this impersonal hospital room, someone paused to reflect on his feelings, to sympathize with his burden with these precious, sparse words "This must be hard for you." Those six words made a difference for him! She was generous, refreshing him with just six words.

GO TO THE ANT.

"Go to the ant...consider its ways and be wise! It has no commander, no overseer or ruler, yet it stores its provisions in summer and gathers its food at harvest" (Proverbs 6:6-8). When we consider the ways of an ant we too can be wise. Besides being on the move to gather their food, ants also work together! One of their unusual ways is how they can support each other during a flood. Fire ants still survive after massive flooding. How? They form a water repellant raft. This was seen when massive flooding took place in South Carolina in October 2015. Homes and businesses were lost and nearly a dozen people lost their lives. Some strange objects were seen in the water after the flooding. Survival rafts were formed by colonies of fire ants. The jaws, legs, and sticky pads of fire ants were used to build living rafts out of their bodies. They can do this in less than two minutes.[26] So, supporting each other is one of the ways of an ant. Supporting each other is a way for us to be wise also.

Supporting each other is another factor in successfully managing diabetes! The two characteristics for success according to the Diabetes Attitudes, Wishes and Needs (DAWN2) Study are a positive outlook and support from family, friends, health care professionals, and other people with diabetes.

In the last chapter, we examined the importance of being optimistic. In this chapter, let's notice how valuable support and kindness are for health and wellness. First, we'll examine examples of kindness like the power of being honest, the comfort a note brings found in a storm's debris, the father who gets a tattoo to mimic his eight year old son's scar left after brain surgery, the teacher who gets a surprise birthday party, a grandson who saves and pays off his grandparent's mortgage, a young man who pays the grocery bill for a frustrated mother, a professor who child-sits a student's children while she takes the final exam, an older couples' car repossessed, an injured teenager who works after his car accident, the unusual result of a liver transplant, kindness to a 97 year old man, a man who jumps from his car to rescue an elderly woman and a man who gives his new boots to a homeless man. Second, we'll examine kindness prescriptions for refreshing and encouraging others.

HONESTY!

What would you do if you found bundles of cash? This happened to "Buzzy" MacCausland, a cabdriver in Boston. He dropped his passenger off at a motel and later he discovered that passenger had left his backpack on the rear seat. In his curiosity he zipped open one of the pockets. What he saw surprised him--he saw cash that was wrapped in bundles. He quickly closed the zipper for he suspected it was "full of cash!"[27]

Three thoughts crossed his mind: keep the treasure, the man could be dangerous and would come after me or take the money to the police. He chose to take the money to the police because he said, "I think it was the right thing to do." "A lot of people said, 'You should have kept it' but I couldn't do that," he explained. Where did he learn such honesty? "That's the way I was brought up. I was told to do the right thing," MacCausland said. The "way of wisdom" teaches this! *"Those who do what is right are guided by their honest lives. But those who aren't faithful are destroyed by their trickery"* (Proverbs 11:3 NIrV).

At the police station the opened backpack revealed bundles of 50's and 100's totaling 187,000 dollars! "I've never seen money like that before. It was quite a sight when they dumped it on the table," he told the news reporters. The police were successful in finding the man, who had been homeless for six months and recently discovered an inheritance.

The police thought so much of the cabbie's honesty that they urged the man to give him a reward. MacCausland thought with a sum like that he might get 500 or 1,000 dollars as a reward, but instead he only got 100 dollars. Who was generous, the cabbie or the inheritance man?

---

*"One person gives freely, yet gains even more; another withholds unduly, but comes to poverty. A generous person will prosper"** (Proverbs 11:24-25).

The man's inheritance was never MacCausland's; he understood this fact. He showed honesty, generosity and gratitude. He was thankful for all the attention his integrity brought with making the news and being complimented by both the police and cab company. Yes, it is true *"Those who are kind benefit themselves"* (Proverbs 11:17).

Watch: "Cabdriver receives $100 dollar reward for returning $187K" at https://www.youtube.com/watch?v=LHikLtaCMOc

*What does prosper mean? The original Hebrew word that is translated "prosper" means "to be fat, grow fat, become fat, become prosperous." In other words, in contrast to skin and bones "prosper" is to be healthy!

COMFORT

"The God of all comfort, who comforts us in all our troubles" (2 Corinthians 1:3-4).

This note—"May God Comfort You"—was found near Ada, Oklahoma in storm debris by a firefighter after some storms. The note not only gave him comfort, but it must have given comfort to many others. He posted it on Facebook and after just a few days it had received 1300 likes. Why so many likes? The reason is because it carries such a meaningful, encouraging message. People face all kinds of challenges in life and need comfort. It may be the loss of possessions from a storm, or the loss of a loved one, one's health, a job or broken relationship. Comfort is needed in those situations and just the thought "May God Comfort You" brings comfort.

Practicing God's wisdom is how comfort so often comes as this example indicates. The phrase under discussion itself is pleasant and can be beneficial to our attitude and health. *"Pleasant words are like honey. They are sweet to the spirit and bring healing to the body"* (Proverbs 16:24). It's amazing what a difference posting a four-word phrase can make. Little is much when kindness is involved.

Kindness brings comfort. One woman in a nursing home dining room was an encourager. She had the biggest smile and seemed so uplifting to everyone around her. People going to their rooms would say good-bye to her from other tables. Everyone in her area seemed to know her. She was a comfort to people in her area of the dining room. As I was observing her she was such a refreshing presence to people around her, including a man who was leaving from our table. He had to say good-bye to her and she said see you tomorrow!

One lady, my mother-in-law made a nice bib with a pocket for her husband there, but she also made two others to be given away. A nurses' aid gave them to two ladies. This little act of kindness brought unexpected comfort, happiness and gratitude. The woman just had to come up to her in the dining room and tell her how much she liked and appreciated the gift! Yes, comfort comes through kindness in a variety of ways and places! *"Blessed is the one who is kind to the needy"* (Proverbs 14:21).

LOVE, LOYALTY, UNDERSTANDING

**"Instead of putting people in their place,
put yourself in their place."**

Do people appreciate understanding saturated with love and loyalty? That is what the way of wisdom teaches. *"Let love and faithfulness never leave you; bind them around your neck, write them on the tablet of your heart. Then you will win favor and a good name in the sight of God and man"* or *"so you will find favor and good understanding in the sight of God and man"* (Proverbs 3:3-4). Compassion, empathy, understanding results from an attitude filled with love and loyalty.

This mindset is reflected in the saying "Instead of putting people in their place, put yourself in their place." That wasn't the attitude expressed by a so-called friend to Job when he said, *"What do you know that we do not know? What insights do you have that we do not have?"* Job 15:9. Harsh and brutal were his comments, especially when considering what his friend was experiencing. Job had faced the loss of almost everything he had—his vast possessions, his ten grown children, his own health, and his wife who was in unbearable grief. How could his friend speak to him in such an uncaring way? Where was his love and loyalty?

It's refreshing when we find love and loyalty flooding someone's life, bringing a thoughtful understanding of another's situation. When confronted with his son's brain tumor and surgery, a father steps forward and shows understanding! Eight-year-old Gabriel Marshall faced a life-threatening brain tumor. The resulting surgery left a large scar, making him feel like a monster. His dad Josh said, "He (Gabriel) was very embarrassed about the scar—he wouldn't even leave the house without something covering his head. He felt like everybody was staring at him and it made him feel like a monster, which broke my heart because to me he's the most beautiful thing."

So, what did Josh do? He decided to get a tattoo to match Gabriel's scar. "I asked him if it would be okay if I went and got his scar tattooed on my head, if that would make him feel better, and he agreed that it would," Josh explained. Gabriel's comment was "Wow that looks so realistic" when Josh came home with the tattoo that looked like his scar. Watch their story at YouTube https://www.youtube.com/watch?v=b6w4c1O94wg

Now with his dad by his side Gabriel has a different perspective. No longer does his scar make him feel like a monster. Instead he feels proud of the scar that shows he was tougher than the tumor that tried to hurt him. He calls it his "battle scar."

This father was saturated with love and loyalty, which resulted in a better understanding of his son! Let's strive to be understanding with others as well. *"Understanding is a fountain of life to those who have it…Good understanding wins favor, but the way of the unfaithful is hard"* (Proverbs 16:22, 13:15).

OPPORTUNITIES FOR KINDNESS

There are certain things in life we consider little and insignificant. They can easily be taken for granted. We should look for trivial things. Count them. List them. Pray about them. They will then overpower a potentially "gloomy day" and turn it "into a bright shiny day!" We can have a good day when we use our hands, see the beauty of flowers and enjoy the aroma and taste of delicious food with gratitude!

Sometimes these little things can grow into the category of big and significant. For example, a casual remark sparked a beautiful act of kindness. "I can't remember the last time I had a birthday cake" was the remark from a high school teacher. He forgot the comment, but his students remembered. They decided to surprise him for his 59th birthday with a birthday cake.

They bought him gifts and a cake with a picture of his favorite feline—Felix. They decorated the classroom with streamers. A video shows how overwhelmed he was with their act of kindness. The students sang "Happy Birthday!" Tears filled his eyes as he walks over to the bookshelf and says, "Thank You." He later said, "It was memorable to say the least. It made me feel good that I have this group of students. These are great kids."

God's wisdom teaches us to look for the good and be thankful. *"He who seeks good finds goodwill, but evil comes to him who searches for it"* (Proverbs 11:27). *"Let the peace of Christ rule in your hearts, since as members of one body you were called to peace. And be thankful"* (Colossians 3:14-15). Look for things that may seem insignificant like the casual comments of people and turn them into something big! The students did. Likewise look for noteworthy things like a birthday cake and be thankful. Thankful were the students for hearing their teacher's casual comment turning it into an opportunity of kindness! Thankful was the teacher for his students celebrating his birthday! Opportunities of kindness come in a variety of ways when we look!

"What is desirable in a man is his kindness"
(Proverbs 19:22 NASB).

Watch: "Students Surprise Their Teacher With His First Birthday Cake in 10 Years" at https://www.youtube.com/watch?v=5a-tQLWEuug

HASTE OR PROLONGED PLANS?

Your phone rings. Your neighbor informs you that a demolition crew is knocking your house down. Can you imagine receiving a phone call like that? A tornado attempted to destroy the house but didn't succeed. Now you're just waiting on insurance and repairs to be scheduled and made when this happens. That bizarre story is a true story that occurred in the Houston area.

So why was a demolition company finishing what the tornado started? They were contracted to tear down a duplex that had sustained irreparable damage from the tornado. The trouble is they were one block off the right location. Google Maps indicated they were at the right address. The demolition company blamed Google Maps and said "not a big deal" and it will all be sorted out by insurance. "Big deal" is a matter of perspective!

What's the lesson? God's wisdom pictures this situation as "missing the way." How is that done? Moving in haste with the wrong information is how! Proverbs 19:2 states, *"It is not good to have zeal without knowledge, nor to be hasty and miss the way."* Instead of just hastily using the Google Maps, why not read the street signs too? Zeal is good when it has knowledge accompanying it. Haste can lead to destructive results, the wrong way, the wrong address.

In contrast is another story from the Houston area. A grandson loves his grandparents so much that he plans to help them pay off their mortgage loan. The amazing part of the story is that he planned to do this since he was in the second grade. He is now a twenty-four-year old college student who just gave his grandparents 15,000 dollars. That was enough to pay their mortgage plus he gave them a trip to the Bahamas. Haste does not characterize this story! Instead there was a well thought out plan to help that took years to accomplish. Stefun Darts said, "Even with this, I could never repay you for what you've done for me." "I sacrificed my teenage and early adulthood of not having fun for this moment. I couldn't stand you going to work at night, some nights I didn't even sleep knowing it shouldn't be like this." We see God's wisdom practiced by this twenty-four-year old. Proverbs 14:22 states, *"Do not those who plot evil go astray? But those who plan what is good find love and faithfulness."* "I couldn't believe it," said Stefun's grandmother. "To have a grandson like that is a blessing." Haste or prolonged plans is the choice![28] *"Wisdom is supreme; therefore get wisdom. Though it cost all you have, get understanding. Esteem her, and she will exalt you; embrace her, and she will honor you* (Proverbs 4:7-8).

THINGS THAT MATTER MOST MUST NEVER BE AT THE MERCY OF THINGS THAT MATTER LEAST

With an internet search for "things that matter" some interesting quotes can be found. What do you think of the following quote? "How wonderful it is that nobody need wait a single moment before starting to improve their world" so said Anne Frank. What is it that really matters? A good question to consider is "How would I want others to remember me when my life is over?" Would you want them to say "He sure knew how to get a nice house and property and live the good life" or "He sure knew how to get what he wanted"? Would those be the things that matter most?

Who knows when our last day will be? Would it make a difference if we were to treat others as though it were their last day? Another internet quote I found was this: "A thousand words will not leave so deep an impression as one deed" so said Henrik Ibsen. An example of one deed took place at a grocery store. Despite being stuck at a busy cash register with no money, a crying baby and a two-hundred-dollar grocery bill she couldn't pay, Jamie-Lynne initially declined an unexpected, generous offer. Matthew was in line behind her and made an offer to pay her bill. She declined and then he insisted "May I?" The only stipulation he had for her was to pay it forward by helping someone else. "Thanking him endlessly through my tears I asked his name and where he worked before parting ways," she recalled.

Several days later she decided to call his workplace to tell his boss what an incredible employee he has. When she called another unexpected response occurred. "I hear crying on the other end of the line and my heart sinks…I just knew something was wrong." She then was told that the night after her groceries were paid by Matthew, he was killed in a car accident. "His boss explained to me how amazing this young man was…what he did for me was just who he was as a person." Matthew's legacy has been posted at Facebook with more than 40,000 comments. His mother read what happened and said, "Hearing what my son did for a complete stranger just one day before he tragically died has been such a gift. My Matthew touched so many and it's amazing that he continues to touch people even after he has left this world. I will miss him terribly…the pain is beyond words. But I know that his legacy will live on."

One person posted "I want my children to know the Matthews of this world. I want them to aspire to be like him and to inspire others to do the same!"[29] Matthew exemplifies God's wisdom in action and demonstrates what really matters in this life. *"Always try to be kind to each other and to everyone else"* (1 Thessalonians 5:15 NIrV).

AN UNUSUAL ACT OF KINDNESS

Where can God's wisdom be found, making an impact? Is it only being used within the walls of a church building? How is it used? Is it used only in songs of praise? Could it be found outside of a college classroom? Solomon wrote 3000 years ago where wisdom can be found and used when he says, *"Wisdom calls aloud in the street, she raises her voice in the public squares; at the head of the noisy streets she cries out, in the gateways of the city she makes her speech"* (Proverbs 1:20-21).

When we look for God's wisdom, we find it. Do you see it in the following headline? "College Professor Babysits Single Mom's Kids So She Can Finish Her Exam." The twenty-eight-year old mother of a four and five-year old was put in a trying situation when her baby sitter didn't show up at the time of her college class exam. So, she decided to bring them with her, letting them play computer games outside the classroom. She said she was filled with "anxiety about it because I knew they weren't going to sit still." And sure enough, it wasn't long before her four-year old boy came knocking on the door. The professor saw him and then discovered her dilemma so he volunteered to watch them so that she wouldn't be distracted while taking the test.[30]

The professor's act of kindness caught her by surprise, but Dr. Krebs insists it was just "common sense", which is often just another way of saying God's wisdom. A friend and fellow student wrote, "Such a kind and caring act committed when the reaction could have been the complete opposite. My heart is warm tonight." *"Being kind to the needy brings happiness"* (Proverbs 14:21 NCV). This act of kindness brought happiness to a friend, the mother and her children and I'm sure to the professor. The professor made quite the impression on at least two young fans who said they had "a lot of fun" with Professor Krebs and want to return to class with their mother. Doesn't that story warm your heart too? Yes, God's wisdom can be found in unusual ways and places and motivates me to want to use wisdom in all facets of my life! Let's use it daily with everyone!

"Do not withhold good from those who deserve it, when it is in your power to act" (Proverbs 3:27).

CAR REPOSSESSED AND KINDNESS?

Jim is in the business of repossessing cars from people who won't pay. What kind of reward has he seen for doing his job? "I've been shot at, ran over, just about everything you can imagine" he said. Would he expect the kind of reaction that Pat gave? "He was wonderful. I mean, he's the kindest man I've ever met in all my life." In fact, she said, "There are good people out there. He's our guardian angel."

God's wisdom says *"Those who are kind reward themselves"* (Proverbs 11:17 NRSV). Mark Twain is remembered for saying, "I can live for two months on a good compliment." Did Jim receive a compliment for taking this couple's car? No, his reward came for what followed a few days later.

Stan and Pat couldn't keep up on their car payments. As Stan was having health issues, they couldn't even make the hundred-dollar payment per month. Not only had they fallen behind on car payments, but they owed the drug store five hundred dollars and couldn't pay their local grocery store as well.

Jim arrived to repossess their car. The only trips they took were to the doctor and drug or grocery store. Pat remarked, "That's about all we ever got to do." Now their means of transportation was gone! When he took the car Pat said, "God, do whatever, whatever you think is best for us. You know, God works in mysterious ways." Jim recalled he didn't expect to see what he saw. This couple reminded him of his own grandparents. His grandparents were no longer living, but he could see them in this couple. When he discovered all that was happening to them, he was really touched (with kindness).

He couldn't just disregard them. He started thinking they were not getting any help as they deserved. His response was the second half of the following proverb: *"It is a sin to despise one's neighbor, but blessed is the one who is kind to the needy"* (Proverbs 14:21). As he left with their car he couldn't get their situation out of his mind. He pulled over and called the bank to ask, "How about I just pay to make their loan current right now?" He set up a GoFundMe account for them. A few days later he brought the car back. It was detailed and polished and even the oil was changed. Plus, it had a frozen turkey on the front seat. Pat couldn't believe her eyes and ears. They "paid the whole thing off." Jim also gave her an envelope with 17,000 dollars extra! Jim was actually using "the way of wisdom" with his kindness. It was at this place in the story that he was called "the kindest man I've ever met" and "a guardian angel."[31] Yes, it is true *"Those who are kind reward themselves"* (Proverbs 11:17 NRSV). *"What is desirable in a man is his kindness"* (Proverbs 19:22 NAS).

Watch: "Couple thankful for repo man who took their car" at https://www.youtube.com/watch?v=8GhFNWMjMPY&index=3&list=PLotzEBRQdc0eX6sErNJED9JuHzJ1vclu_

HARD WORK, GOODWILL AND GENEROSITY

"The lazy will not get what they want, but those who work hard will" (Proverbs 13:4 NCV).

How would you spot a generous, determined person? Would he go to work wearing both a neck brace and an arm sling for injuries from a recent car accident? Jakeem is a high school student who works part-time at Chick-fil-A near Indianapolis.[32] His manager strongly suggested he go back home when he walked into work wearing his brace and sling. Instead, he insisted on working! Why? He needed the money, not for himself, to buy gifts and food for the homeless. In fact, his father related that he often buys food and shares it with those in need on his way home from work! Helping others less fortunate was his focus even after being injured in a car accident. What a commendable attitude!

On that same day, the drive-thru was so backed up that one man went inside. To his surprise, he saw Jakeem at the cash register wearing his neck brace and arm sling while helping customers. Cameron wrote, "We sneeze too hard and decide to call in (sick), but he's working like nothing's wrong...I was amazed he's still working despite his condition." That is when he had to ask what happened and why he was working. Cameron was so impressed with Jakeem's caring attitude that he set up a GoFundMe to help with his benevolent efforts. The goal was 2500 dollars. At last count, more than 43,000 dollars had been donated by 1,700 people, which is an average of 25 dollars per person!

Not only was Cameron impressed by Jakeem, but Jakeem was impressed by what Cameron did. He was very thankful and said "I always had it in my heart to give back to people." Look what his example of goodwill brought—an overwhelming flood of funds to help. These funds would benefit many people with food and clothing! What a good person like Jakeem did is well illustrated in the "wisdom" of Proverbs 21:25-26. "Lazy people's desire for sleep will kill them, because they refuse to work. All day long they wish for more, but good people give without holding back." "The only thing they asked us was to remember to help the poor—something I really wanted to do" (Galatians 2:10).—The Apostle Paul

Watch: "Chick-fil-A employee responds to viral photo showing him working through injury" at https://www.youtube.com/watch?v=1l4TPflUINs

KINDNESS IS DESIRABLE

"What is desirable in a man is his kindness" (Proverbs 19:22 NAS). Kind treatment is nice and usually wanted! We see it in many ways. Kindness should be shown in how the poor, the needy, and even animals or pets are treated. *"Whoever is kind to the poor lends to the LORD, and he will reward them for what they have done...Blessed is the one who is kind to the needy...The righteous care for the needs of their animals"* (Proverbs 19:17, 14:21, 12:10). Sometimes we see kindness expressed in unbelievable ways especially when a kind act gives life to another! Heather Krueger said, "I think first of all that it shows everyone, when all you hear is negativity, that there really are sincerely kind people out there."

Suffering from liver failure Heather was in desperate need of a liver transplant. Her transplant did happen, but in an unusual way. Her cousin worked for the Village of Frankfort in Illinois. He was telling a co-worker about her urgent need. That's when Chris overheard the conversation. He's the kind of city code enforcement officer who looks for unusual ways to solve complaints instead of just writing a ticket. For example, when complaints were made of a ninety-year-old lady's house needing repairs, he got thirty volunteers who helped with those repairs. When Chris heard of Heather's need, he decided to see if he could be a donor. He said, "When I heard about her, I just thought I would want someone to help me. I spent four years in the Marine Corps and learned there never to run away from anything." Surprisingly he was a donor match! When he discovered the good news, he had to share it and called Heather to let her know. He had never talked to her or met her. Of course, she was thrilled with the news. When she got off the phone she was so excited that she ran down the hallway telling her mother. They both had tears of disbelief! She admitted, "I had never even met this man before."

She had her successful transplant, but that is not the end of the story. She attended a wedding last October. The wedding was hers. A groomsman was her cousin who was telling of her situation at work. Chris was honored to attend also, but as the groom! He had never intended for this wedding to happen. Before their surgery he didn't know her and she didn't know him. He literally gave her more than half of his liver while a year and a half later, in a sense, she gave him her heart.[33] This story is truly a definition for Proverbs 19:22, isn't it! *"What is desirable in a man is his kindness."* Watch "A stranger's selfless gift leads to love" at https://www.youtube.com/watch?v=JCsrWoC2oDg

---

"A generous person will prosper; whoever refreshes others will be refreshed" (Proverbs 11:25). *"Do to others as you would have them do to you"* (Luke 6:31).

TWO SIDES OF A STORY

A story may have two sides. That's why it is better to wait before coming to a conclusion. Waiting will bring a better understanding. *"The person who tells one side of a story seems right, until someone else comes and asks questions…Patient people have great understanding"* (Proverbs 18:17, 14:29 NCV).

Waiting can bring good acts! For example, in the recent World Series between the Chicago Cubs and Cleveland Indians a 97-year-old fan and World War II veteran, Jim Schlegel, has been waiting for his team. He's waited since the time of President Truman. Unlike most people he saw them play in Wrigley field in 1945 just after coming home from the war. He's never seen them win a series because the last time that happened was when the first Ford Model T's were coming off the assembly lines, which was in 1908.

Of course, this avid fan hoped to go this time, but there was only one problem—the cost. In 1945 a ticket cost seven-dollars and fifty cents. Now tickets were going as high as 21,000 dollars. Jim's granddaughter wasn't going to let cost keep him from going. She wanted to do all she could to help. She set up a "GoFundMe" page to raise $10,000 in hopes to purchase a ticket. It took only one day to reach the goal because of the kindness of many people. The other side of the story, however, is that the funds were not needed. A search for a perfect Cubs fan was conducted by Marcus Lemonis, the host of a TV show. When he heard the story of Jim, he knew the perfect fan was found. Contact was made with the family and two front-row seat tickets were given to Jim for the third game. What happened to the more than $11,000 given on the "GoFundMe" page? Was it kept by the family? No, again we see kindness and generosity at work; we see the other side of the story. The family made plans to donate the funds to the Purple Heart Foundation. (This foundation helps soldiers with emotional, medical, financial needs and more.)

We see in this story the way of wisdom that includes patience, kindness and generosity. *"I guide you in the way of wisdom and lead you along straight paths...A generous person will prosper; whoever refreshes others will be refreshed"* (Proverbs

4:11). Generosity refreshes people—both giver and receiver. The other side of the story is Jim was encouraged, but many veteran soldiers will be as well. Jim was able to go with his son, and the Cubs won the game!

Watch: "97-Year-Old Chicago Fan Sees Cubs In World Series For First Time Since 1945" at https://www.youtube.com/watch?v=WtDTqF74nRs or "97-year-old World War ii vet cubs fan gets a world series surprise" at https://www.youtube.com/watch?v=aV60jbv-sSQ

MAN JUMPS FROM CAR AND RESCUES ELDERLY WOMAN

God's wisdom states, *"He who despises his neighbor sins, but blessed is he who is kind to the needy"* (Proverbs 14:21). Being kind to the needy could include a needy neighbor. Kindness is important to God. Another way in which kindness is expressed is by rescuing people. *"Rescue those being led away to death; hold back those staggering toward slaughter"* (Proverbs 24:11). Some noteworthy examples of rescue have been in the news lately.

Can you imagine sitting at a railroad crossing with the warning gates down? Sure, you can, but also with an elderly woman trying to cross the tracks? The woman seems petrified on the tracks with a speeding locomotive approaching and horn blaring. In this situation timing was everything because Jon leaped from his car, quickly moved under the gates and grabbed the woman by the arms, pulling her off the tracks. Without a split second to spare the train missed them by inches. Jon Mango's dashboard camera recorded it all.

Mango said. "She actually stopped because she was scared, so then I tried grabbing her arm and then really tried pulling her. She was having a lot of trouble." This rescue was dangerous since the train missed their bodies by inches. His sister thought what he did was just characteristic of her brother. She said, "This act is so reflective of who he is as a person. Just a genuine selfless human always wanting to help others," she wrote on Facebook. That should be characteristic of us all according to God's wisdom. Nothing good is accomplished when one just observes the needs of others. Nothing good would have happened for that elderly woman if Jon had just stayed in his car. Action was needed and a benevolent act was done. This is the way of God's wisdom. *"Those who give to the poor will lack nothing, but those who close their eyes to them receive many curses...If you refuse to listen to the cry of the poor, your own cry for help will not be heard"* (Proverbs 28:27, 21:13).

God's wisdom also *states "There is a time for everything, and a season for every activity under the heavens"* (Ecclesiastes 3:1). This was a time, a dramatic time, to save the woman from the speeding train. Dramatic times like that don't occur every day, but times to rescue people from discouragement do. Research indicates that singing brings emotional and physical benefits. We didn't need the research recently when seventeen of us went to sing to those mostly confined to their homes. We were rescuing them from discouragement. Encouragement, smiles of joy and expressions of gratitude followed. *"Anyone who is having troubles should pray. Anyone who is happy should sing praises"* (James 5:13). Let's strive to rescue people from difficulties each day. That is what God desires!

"Encourage one another daily, as long as it is called "Today," so that none of you may be hardened by sin's deceitfulness" Hebrews 3:13.

Watch: "Man Jumps From Car, Saves Elderly Woman from Oncoming NJ Transit Train" https://www.youtube.com/watch?v=COLR30cdRAQ

BOOTS

"Produce fruit in keeping with repentance" (Luke 3:8). When people repent they are to change their lives, that is, produce fruit. People may next ask, *"What should we do then?"* John gave examples by saying, *"Anyone who has two shirts should share with the one who has none"* (Luke 3:10-11). In other words, be kind and compassionate to people in need.

On a Chicago transit train, this teaching of John was vividly practiced. The weather was cold and to escape that cold a homeless man found refuge on the train. A woman seated across from him noticed the old, limp and tattered shoes on his feet. They were gym shoes with the backs folded down, like slip-ons. Several layers of socks were on his feet to keep them warm, but she still saw blood seeping through.

All of a sudden, a man sitting nearby asked him what size shoes he wore. His size was the same as this stranger's brand new two hundred sixty-dollar winter boots. He began to unlace and handed them to the man. He opened his suitcase, took out a pair of socks and gave them to the man. In the end he put on some older shoes from his suitcase.

Shocked, but appreciative, was the homeless man's reaction! The woman witnessing this interaction was pleasantly surprised by the kindness shown. She took pictures of the man receiving the boots and posted the incident on Facebook. The episode went "viral" within a short time, receiving more than 13,000 shares and 26,000 likes.[34]

Doesn't this story remind you of the instruction John gave? This kind man expressed that he doesn't judge people in difficult situations but often helps the homeless by giving them clothing or supplies. *"It is a sin to despise one's neighbor, but blessed is the one who is kind to the needy"* (Proverbs 14:21).

Watch: "Good Samaritan Gives Homeless Man Winter Boots off His Feet" at https://www.youtube.com/watch?v=vwCula-S-kY

VOLUNTEER PRESCRIPTION: RANDOM ACTS OF KINDNESS

Aristotle surmised that the essence of life is "To serve others and do good." Hundreds of years before Aristotle Solomon wrote, *"Blessed is the one who is kind to the needy...whoever is kind to the needy honors God...Whoever is kind to the poor lends to the LORD, and he will reward them for what they have done...The generous will themselves be blessed, for they share their food with the poor"* (Proverbs 14:21,31, 19:17, 22:9). This is the way of God's wisdom.

Research indicates benefits of volunteering like better mental health and lower rates of depression. Another benefit is lower blood pressure. This may be a result of lifestyle though. People who volunteer probably take better care of themselves with exercise and healthy eating.[35] Volunteering can be a building block of that healthy lifestyle. The Mayo Clinic lists six health benefits of volunteering: decreases the risk of depression, gives a sense of purpose, helps people stay physically and mentally active, may reduce stress levels and live longer as well as meet people.

They also provide many opportunities to volunteer as do other hospitals. People can serve as greeters, giving assistance with patient room information and directions; others transport patients and their items. They assist in surgery and Critical Care waiting rooms. Blankets, sweaters and hats are made and given to newborn babies and cancer patients. These are just some of the ways volunteering is done in hospitals.[36]

Churches have ways to volunteer also. Ours has a clothing house to assist people in the community in need of children's clothing, clothing after a fire or some tragedy. Clothing from the community is given and separated by size and quality to keep or discard. Meals are prepared for grieving families after a funeral or taken to people's homes who have been sick or released from the hospital. We also provide a Diabetes Support Group.

The following is a list of ways we can all informally volunteer. They are acts of kindness called "Pass It On." "Give a flower. Eat lunch with someone new. Listen with your heart. Visit a sick friend. Clean a neighbor's walk. Offer a hug. Give an unexpected gift. Make a new friend. Pick up litter. Say "hello." Call a lonely person. Open a door. Help carry a load. Plant a tree. Pass a kindness on. Buy someone's meal. Cheer up a friend. Thank a teacher. Give blood. Read to a child. Do one kind act every day. Leave a thank you note. Offer your seat. Tip generously. Be tolerant.

Let another go first. Bake cookies for emergency workers. Tutor a student. Give a compliment. Pay the next driver's toll. Lend a hand. Give a balloon to a child. Offer a ride. Celebrate the day. Respect others. Encourage a child. Walk a dog. Do a favor. Forgive mistakes. Drive courteously. Share a smile."[37]

SUPPORT PRESCRIPTION

When I was recovering from back surgery, a laminectomy in 1988, I was kept in a wing of a large hospital just for patients with diabetes. I was thirty-five. During my stay of ten days I discovered five people who were already blind from diabetes, four were younger than me and one about five years older. It took me almost thirty years to realize how serious this disease is. I saw it. Two years before this I had a massive hemorrhage in my right eye. So, I resolved to help people, to help them feel better every day, to support them so that they wouldn't have to face such devastating results. That decision helped me get better control of my own diabetes as well.

In the fall of 1992, I started a diabetes support group at the Good Samaritan Hospital in Kearney, Nebraska. For the first meeting thirty-five attended. I introduced myself and for the next several years I gave encouraging support to those who attended, helping hundreds of people. For the last twenty-five years I've continued to facilitate either hospital or community support groups where ever I've lived.

Many people will not admit they have diabetes or any chronic disease. Their disease is private, their secret. What is missed with that attitude? The opportunity to not only help others, but to help themselves as well. Eventually the hospital in

Kearney, Nebraska hired a Certified Diabetes Educator. One day I received a call from her, telling me there was a noncompliant patient with Type 1 diabetes in the hospital. Would I visit him? I agreed. He would not cooperate even putting the sheets over his head when they entered his room. When I asked to enter his room, identifying myself as a fellow Type 1, he invited me in and opened up to me.

We talked about the challenges we were both facing. He was finding great difficulty in keeping his blood sugar under control. He had never had any support or encouragement. His mom was not helpful. Friends of hers had even influenced him to drink. So, after he was released from the hospital he attended the support group meetings. We also met on a weekly basis. I shared portions from a book called "Diabetes: A Guide to Living Well" by Dr. Gary Arsham. Dr. Arsham was diagnosed with Type 1 diabetes when he was ten. Unlike today, there were few books available for people with diabetes in 1994. So, in a sense, he became part of our weekly meetings. People need encouragement. Randy started doing better with his blood sugar levels, but he already had kidney failure. He started on Peritoneal Dialysis.

Not only did we use the diabetes guide book, but we looked at encouraging Proverbs like *"The fear of the LORD is the beginning of wisdom, and knowledge of the Holy One is understanding. For through wisdom your days will be many, and years will be added to your life. If you are wise, your wisdom will reward you"* (Proverbs 9:10-12). He started coming to Bible class. When he started his mom wanted to know why in the world he was doing that. He said because he had never tried it before. He was trying a lot of new things like routinely checking his blood sugar. He wanted to see if attending Bible class would make a difference. And it did! One day after eating lunch together, as we travelled toward my office, we saw a lawn that really needed mowing. The person who lived there was a widow woman, a recluse whose husband had died in World War 2. I casually said we should just go mow her lawn. After saying that I went on a trip out of state. When I got back I discovered Randy had taken his own mower in the trunk of his car and mowed the whole lawn, taking the cuttings to the dump yard. I asked if she ever said anything to him. She only said, "What are you doing?" No, thanks, no gratitude! Randy was practicing God's wisdom. *"Blessed is the one who is kind to the needy"* (Proverbs 14:21). That is the kind of behavior a Christian should have. So, a few days later he became a Christian, being baptized into Christ (read Acts 22:16, Galatians 3:27, Romans 6:3-4).

Randy was on a kidney transplant list and not long after this wonderful news arrived—a kidney and pancreas. When he received that pancreas, he was no longer in the community of diabetics. This good news was countered with bad news because within a few weeks he was in a car/train wreck. The train won. He was flown to Omaha with a broken femur, ribs, arm and severe trauma to his head. He was in rehab for months. How did he stay encouraged during those weeks of therapy? He focused on good things. He said just as Paul walked on water as long as he kept his eyes on Jesus, (it was actually Peter), I keep my eyes on Jesus. Here is a question he asked me. What is the most rewarding thing about your job? "What is most rewarding" I said "is when I see people encouraged and helped!"

Look for people you can encourage. For example, start a walking club! One woman at our diabetes support group knew she needed to start walking. She needed motivation! She asked at a support group meeting if anyone would meet her at the park to help her get started. Three people volunteered. But instead of just three showing up, twelve did! Can you imagine how it would be to show up to walk and have about a dozen others there to help you get started? It would be encouraging and motivating! I've discovered that when I look for people I can encourage and support, they've helped me too! Those who showed up to help her get started walking, walked too. So, in a sense, she was helping them, also. When we look for others to support, we too will be encouraged! Blessed and refreshed will result just as Jesus and Solomon said: *"It is more blessed to give than to receive... A generous person will prosper; whoever refreshes others will be refreshed"* (Acts 20:35, Proverbs 11:25).

IMITATE JESUS PRESCRIPTION

"A student is not above his teacher, but everyone who is fully trained will be like his teacher." –Jesus

Remember a time when you felt grateful for something that someone did for you! That "something" is usually meaningful and significant. When one person shared the details of what others did for him, he described them as life changing for his life was literally saved. "That's not all they saved," he said. "They saved my family the pain of losing me. They saved my little sister's big brother. They saved me the time with my family that I would've never gotten." Does that sound significant? Does that sound meaningful? How was he saved?

Firefighters saved him. He was on the second floor of an apartment complex that was ablaze like a bonfire. This fire was huge! After climbing the ladder and going through the window a firefighter had found him unconscious. He awoke three days later in ICU at the hospital. Nurses told him what happened. He spent the next week in the hospital recovering. His story, and the remembrance of what they had done for him, motivated him.

Four years later a stranger arrived at the fire station for a "ride along" (a program designed for observation of a day in the life of a firefighter). At first no one recognized him until fifteen minutes later he told the major who he was—the person they carried out of an apartment fire four-years before and saved his life! They had given him a great desire! His desire was save others' lives! He had decided to earn his firefighter's degree.[38]

Two thousand years ago another man's life was saved. No one would have anything to do with him. He was an outcast because he was a hated tax collector. No one would expect the rabbi, the teacher, to go to his home and eat with him. His name was Zacchaeus and since he was so short he climbed a sycamore-fig tree to see Jesus among the crowd. *"When Jesus reached the spot, he looked up and said to him, 'Zacchaeus, come down immediately. I must stay at your house today' So, he came down at once and welcomed him gladly."* Then we find him saying something very interesting. His life was being changed by Jesus. Jesus coming to his home was already motivating kindness in him. He said, *"Look, Lord! Here and now I give half of my possessions to the poor, and if I have cheated anybody out of anything, I will pay back four times the amount"* (Luke 19:5-6, 8). Zacchaeus was showing he was a changed man, a man of compassion. Jesus had saved this outcast's life. Would this be the "something" Zacchaeus could remember with gratitude? When we think back on events that others have done for us, it brings out the best in us. It happened to the man saved by firefighters and it happened to Zacchaeus. *"For the Son of Man came to seek and to save the lost"* (Luke 19:10).

Jesus had a reputation for being compassionate and kind toward people. He cared about people. When he looked at people he pictured them as being harassed and helpless like sheep without a shepherd. He saw hurting people! *"He said to his disciples, 'The harvest is plentiful but the workers are few. Ask the Lord of the harvest, therefore, to send out workers into his harvest field'"* (Matthew 9:37-38.) He saw the need for more kind, compassionate workers!

Paul, who described himself as a persecutor and a violent man, the worst of sinners became a zealous, bold, kind, compassionate man. He writes, *"Christ Jesus came into the world to save sinners—of whom I am the worst"* (1 Timothy 1:15). He describes patience and kindness as attributes of love, which is what Jesus had for him (1 Corinthians 13:4). Jesus' love for him, his mercy and kindness changed his life from violence to kindness (read Titus 3:4-5). Treating people as Jesus did was his desire. In fact, he wrote, *"Be imitators of me as I am of Christ"* (1 Corinthians 11:1). He describes Jesus' disciples as *"God's handiwork, created in Christ Jesus to do good works"* (Ephesians 2:10). Being *"devoted to doing what is good"* is one reason he says he was saved, being delivered from his sins (Titus 3:8). Grasping the depth of Jesus love for him compelled him to live, not for himself, but for Jesus—to live a life of love (2 Corinthians 5:14, Ephesians 5:2). While he was a violent man, hunting down disciples of Jesus to force them to deny their loyalty to Jesus or be imprisoned or even put to death, he was struck blind (Acts 26:11). He was on the road to Damascus when a bright light from heaven blinded him. Jesus spoke to him saying, *"Saul, Saul, why do you persecute me?" "Who are you, Lord?" Saul asked. "I am Jesus, whom you are persecuting," he replied. "Now get up and go into the city, and you will be told what you must do"* (Acts 9:4-6). So, he went into Damascus. blind, praying and fasting for three days, Ananias, a disciple of Jesus came to him and said, *"And now what are you waiting for? Get up, be baptized and wash your sins away, calling on his name"* (Acts 22:16). This was the moment he was saved, becoming a disciple of Jesus.

He could see again, but he saw life in a different way. He was given a new life. He was a new creation. *"If anyone is in Christ, the new creation has come: The old has gone, the new is here"* (2 Corinthians 5:17). His sins were washed away—all the havoc and harm he had done to people was forgiven! He was a changed man. Instead of persecuting people he began telling people how much Jesus loved them as he lived a life of love himself. He said, *"I showed you that by this kind of hard work we must help the weak, remembering the words the Lord Jesus himself said: 'It is more blessed to give than to receive'"* (Acts 20:35).

When he told people how to become compassionate, kind disciples of Jesus he tied it directly to what Jesus had done for them. *"Or don't you know that all of us who were baptized into Christ Jesus were baptized into his death? We were therefore buried with him through baptism into death in order that, just as Christ was raised from the dead through the glory of the Father, we too may live a new life"* (Romans 6:3-4). And just how much does he say Jesus loves us? *You see, at just the right time, when we were still powerless, Christ died for the ungodly. Very rarely will anyone die for a righteous person, though for a good person someone might possibly dare to die. But God demonstrates his own love for us in this: While we were still sinners, Christ died for us"* (Romans 5:6-8). A righteous person is one who is just and fair, whereas, a good person is one who is just, fair and generous.

Paul, however, is saying we are all in the ungodly category and yet Jesus was still willing to die for us. That makes us in Jesus' view most valuable people! So, the apostle John writes, *"This is how we know what love is: Jesus Christ laid down his life for us"* (1 John 3:16). In summarizing Jesus' life, Peter said *"he went around doing good"* (Acts 10:38). Let's do the same!

CHAPTER THREE

The Power of Motivation

"The appetite of laborers works for them; their hunger drives them on" (Proverbs 16:26).

I know there are so many things I need to do to get healthy, but I just can't muster up enough willpower to do what I need to do! It seems like some people are given willpower and others don't have the gift. What am I to do?

Some view willpower as the key to getting things done. One person in a doctor's waiting room read an article about how to get things done. The article promoted willpower as the way to accomplish things! He read, "Forget about motivation. Just do it. Exercise, lose weight, test your blood sugar, or whatever. Do it without motivation and then guess what. After you start doing the thing, that's when the motivation comes and makes it easy for you to keep on doing it." That may be true when we think of motivation as just an emotion or a feeling rather than a reason or motive for doing something.

It's been taught to act loving toward someone even when you don't feel loving and eventually the result is the feeling of love. That all sounds good, but where do we get the willpower to start acting? According to God's wisdom, willpower starts with motivation. *"The appetite of laborers works for them; their hunger drives them on"* (Proverbs 16:26). *"All a man's ways seem innocent to him, but motives are weighed by the LORD"* (Proverbs 16:2). Motivation is important and drives a person on! Notice the factor of motivation in the following six examples.

WILLPOWER OR MOTIVATION?

Lose weight. Move more. Practice daily discipline. Run a half marathon in three hours, fourteen minutes. Lose fifteen pounds was doctor prescribed for health concerns. She ran in the University of Pittsburgh Medical Center's Half Marathon run with forty less pounds than she had several months earlier, not just fifteen less.

Chris said she is my inspiration. "I use her courage to give myself courage. If she can do this, then I can do this." Why is courage needed and who is she? Her name is Rebekah. She is the one who lost forty pounds and ran a half marathon. Was willpower the secret for her accomplishments or was it motivation?

When doctors told Rebekah, she had to lose fifteen pounds she reacted. "Admittedly, I was really angry that two individual surgeons would have the audacity to say such a thing, but they were right," Rebekah said. "My actual thought was, 'I'm too fat to save my friend's life.'" There is the key for what she did—saving a friend's life.[39]

One day as she was viewing what friends were saying on Facebook she noticed a message that grabbed her attention and wouldn't let go. It was a message from a former coworker, Chris, who was suffering from chronic kidney disease. His future looked bleak. Within six months to a year, he would require a kidney transplant, or worse, dialysis. That sad news is what motivated or compelled Rebekah to have the willpower to lose weight in order to donate a kidney. Let's look for motivation that will help us get things done too!

"For Christ's love compels us" or "urges us on" (2 Corinthians 5:14). "Being rooted and established in love, may have power...to grasp how wide and long and high and deep is the love of Christ" (Ephesians 3:17-18).

PRIORITY: WHEN YOU HAVE TO MOW THE LAWN, YOU HAVE TO MOW THE LAWN

"There is a time for everything, and a season for every activity under the heavens" (Ecclesiastes 3:1). There is a season for everything, including the season for mowing lawns. Rain storms and sunshine encourage the grass. The growing grass has no concern for our schedules; it will continue to get taller. If we wait too long to cut the grass, the mowing will really become an unwanted chore. One man in Alberta, Canada, knew he had a busy schedule. When he had the opportunity to mow, he mowed. There is nothing unusual about this story yet. However, the headline for this story gives a different image. "As this tornado touched down last week in Alberta, Canada, one guy had a more pressing matter at hand than taking cover." And, the picture shows him

mowing as a threatening tornado is spinning behind him. He was so determined—when you have to mow, you have to mow! What would you do? This was the best time for him to mow, but the tornado tried to interrupt his schedule. What was he to do? He admitted, "I would say halfway through the mowing process a tornado started forming, and I just kept my eye on it." This man, originally from South Africa where tornadoes are rare, apparently didn't realize the danger of a tornado. In fact, in an interview that danger was stated to him and he just smiled. He said it was the first time he had ever seen one, and his wife had to take the picture of him mowing with the tornado in the background to send to family back home. Why did he continue to mow instead of take shelter? He said his kids had many events to attend that weekend and he had to get the lawn cut then!

God's wisdom is written to guide us for health and well-being. *"They (proverbs) are life to those who find them and health to one's whole body"* (Proverbs 4:22). There are proverbs that warn us to take refuge when we see something dangerous. When I recently went to the grand opening of a new grocery store, I was surprised to see so many people who looked unhealthy. Could the advertising of "junk food" bargains have had anything to do with that? *"A prudent man sees danger and takes refuge, but the simple keep going and suffer for it"* (Proverbs 22:3).

There are proverbs that teach about setting priorities. *"Finish your outdoor work and get your fields ready; after that, build your house"* (Proverbs 24:27). This proverb recommends putting first things first. In other words, secure an income before getting in debt up to your "eyeballs." The image of the man mowing with a tornado in the background is a perfect picture of priorities.

Which comes first? "Am I doing things right?" Or "am I doing the right things?" Let's stay healthy by doing the right things. He was motivated. He had things he wanted to do with his family that weekend. Yes, he was motivated but let's combine that with doing the right things at the right time too!

Watch: "Keeping my eye on it': Man mows lawn as tornado approaches at **https://www.youtube.com/ watch?v=BKjcjti6DkM**

EXCEPTIONAL

Exceptional is not a word that most people hear about themselves. You're nothing exceptional may be as close as some people come to hearing those words. What is it that makes a person exceptional? Is it looks, brains, money, possessions or achievements? To God each person is special and significant. It doesn't matter if they have money.

"Whoever oppresses the poor shows contempt for their Maker, but whoever is kind to the needy honors God" (Proverbs 14:31).

Each person can show the value of others with kindness. We are instructed with God's wisdom to do this even with animals. *"The righteous care for the needs of their animals, but the kindest acts of the wicked are cruel"* (Proverbs 12:10). Kindness is expected! Did you hear about the German Shephard in the news? Meet Quasimodo, the dog with the short spine.[40]

A shelter for large breed dogs with special needs is housing him. Some have named him after the "Hunchback of Notre

Dame" character. They are being kind to this pup. Quasi is one of only 13 known dogs in the world with short spine syndrome. "Born different but never knowing any other way, he seeks to please the people who have shown him kind hands and warm hearts," Sara Anderson, the shelter manager said. God's wisdom is being practiced with this dog. So, is it intelligence or looks that makes one exceptional?

You've heard of Fanny Crosby (1820-1915)! We sing some of the 8000 hymns she wrote like "All the Way My Savior Leads Me" or "Blessed Assurance." At six weeks old she had an eye infection that was incorrectly treated causing blindness. As a teenager at the New York Institution for the Blind, she was already showing her talent as a writer. "My friends had nearly spoiled me with their praises," she wrote later. "I began to feel my own importance as a poet a little too much."

The superintendent summoned her to his office one day. "Fanny," he said, "I am sorry you have allowed yourself to be carried by what others have said about your verses." He warned her to "shun flattery." He then said something she never forgot. "Remember that whatever talent you possess belongs wholly to God that you ought to give Him the credit for all that you do." A few years later, she wrote "To God Be the Glory." *"He has told you what he wants from you: to do what is right to other people, love being kind to others, and live humbly, obeying your God"* (Micah 6:8). *"So whether you eat or drink or whatever you do, do it all for the glory of God"* (1 Corinthians 10:31). What is exceptional? It has nothing to do with power, prestige, possession or popularity. To treat others with kindness, giving glory to God is what is truly exceptional and motivational for doing the right things!

LONGEVITY

Willard Scott, weatherman on the Today show, was best known not only for his weather forecasts but also for greeting those turning one hundred years old throughout the United States. He started this practice way back in 1983. Turning to the age of 100 grabbed peoples' attention back then and it still does. Even more significant is to be the oldest person in a state. For Oklahoma that person is Mary Manek Erbin (my mother-in-law's cousin). She turned 109 years old on August 15. She was born to Ukrainian immigrants north of Harrah in Indian Territory before statehood.

We all desire to live a longer life. When she was asked about her long life she expressed several ideas like never smoking or drinking. She worked even into her eighties. She remembered picking cotton and working very hard when she was younger. Her grandson said she was picking blackberries when she was in her eighties. "We all picked, but she out-picked all of us. We picked by the quart and she was picking by the bucket." More than anything else, she said that all you have to do is live an honest, dedicated life and trust in God to live a long life.

Documented research has been done to locate where more people live to be a hundred than anywhere else—the island of Okinawa. Honesty and hard work are two characteristics that are attributed to the islanders' longevity. In fact, the word "retirement" does not exist in the traditional Okinawan dialect. Many people are still farming even up to the age of 100. Honesty and support for others are so prevalent that you could leave your wallet on the sidewalk in Okinawa and expect it to still be there the next day.

Honesty and hard work are two characteristics that 109-year-old Mary also expressed. What does God's wisdom say about longevity? *"For through wisdom your days will be many, and years will be added to your life. If you are wise, your wisdom will reward you"* (Proverbs 9:11-12). We shouldn't be surprised that hard work and honesty are the teachings of God's wisdom. *"Good people will be guided by honesty; dishonesty will destroy those who are not trustworthy...Wise words bring many benefits, and hard work brings rewards"* (Proverbs 11:3 NCV, 12:14 NLT). Yes, God's wisdom works just as well in Indian Territory (and later in Oklahoma) as it does in Okinawa. *"Does not wisdom call out?...To you, O people, I call out; I raise my voice to all mankind"* (Proverbs 8:1, 4). Let us use that wisdom to motivate us to live a long life.

TEACHING LONGEVITY

Have you ever noticed how TV commercials promote an idea of "the fountain of youth?" I recently watched a commercial that went on and on and about the removal of "crepe" skin. By using this product, one could regain the looks of youth! People may focus on extending their lives from so-called "fountain of youth" products. What most people overlook, however, is God's wisdom. *"For through wisdom your days will be many, and years will be added to your life"* (Proverbs 9:11).

I took a graduate college class on what is known as the Wisdom Literature of the Old Testament (Job, Psalms, Proverbs, and Ecclesiastes). This unique class started at eight o'clock in the morning. No one was ignored; each student was welcomed to class. The teacher walked around the class, wishing good morning to each student and offering a delicious home-made cookie. After the offer of cookies, songs would be sung based upon Old Testament passages. We sang newly composed songs (this was 1980) like *"The Steadfast Love of the Lord"* (Lamentations 3) or *"Unto Thee, O Lord"* (Psalm 25). Then what followed were his excellent insights and applications of Psalms, Proverbs or Job.

This teacher was Dr. John T. Willis. He has recently retired at the age of eighty-three after sixty-one years of teaching! By welcoming us to class and giving us cookies, he was practicing several principles of God's wisdom. Offering a few cookies before each class, is that generosity? God's wisdom gives this principle on how little amounts can add up to generosity. *"Whoever gathers money little by little makes it grow"* (Proverbs 13:11). It's been estimated he gave nearly one million cookies to more than 16,000 students during his teaching career. Wisdom says, *"The generous will themselves be blessed, for they share their food with the poor...blessed is the one who is kind to the needy"* (Proverbs 22:9, 14:21). This respected professor gave his students value with his thoughtfulness to each one. That is the kind of class you wanted to attend! The singing, in which we participated at each class, was another principle of wisdom. *"Worship the LORD with gladness; come before him with joyful songs"* (Psalm 100:2). And yes, teaching is another wisdom principle. *"I instruct you in the way of wisdom and lead you along straight paths...Hold on to instruction, do not let it go; guard it well, for it is your life"* (Proverbs 4:11,13). He formally instructed us in wisdom, as well as by example.

Longevity comes with the practice of wisdom. (Proverbs are observations of what usually happens to people, not promises of what will happen with no exceptions.)

"The fear of the LORD adds length to life, but the years of the wicked are cut short" (Proverbs 10:27).

Let's determine to practice generosity and kindness with people. That is God's wisdom—the fountain of youth! *"The teaching of the wise is a fountain of life, turning a person from the snares of death"* (Proverbs 13:14). Getting this fountain of life to others is motivational.

SURPRISE PARTY ON HER 90TH BIRTHDAY

The following is a news headline that caught my attention: "Hospital Throws America's Oldest Working Nurse a Surprise Party On Her 90th Birthday."[41] Her name is Florence "See See" Rigney. She has been faithfully helping patients for over six decades. She is currently still working as a nurse at Tacoma General Hospital in Washington. Last Friday she celebrated her 90th birthday and she got a surprise birthday party. She is America's oldest working nurse. She was greeted by hospital staff with birthday wishes, flowers, and a letter of congratulations from the governor. As she thanked them for the well wishes, she could hardly hold back tears. She was genuinely touched by the recognition she received for just a birthday. She even expressed that fact that it was hard for her to believe she was turning ninety. In the video it was obvious that she has a good relationship with the staff. She was a very vibrant and animated ninety-year old with the celebration! "The oldest working nurse in the United States turns 90 and still going!" https://www.youtube.com/watch?v=9JtriJkFmm0 "Inspiring America: Meet America's Oldest Working Nurse | NBC Nightly News" https://www.youtube.com/watch?v=hrFFbARY-KQ

I see God's wisdom being displayed in several ways from this event. First, she is fortunate to have good health at her age and with that health be able to continue to help or bless others. Her occupation demands that she focus on helping others. Do you think during those decades of service each patient has been amiable and cooperative? There are many passages that teach us to serve and be kind to those in need. These passages talk about the poor, but people can be poor financially as well as be poor in health. *"Being kind to the poor is like lending to the Lord; he will reward you for what you have done...The generous will themselves be blessed, for they share their food with the poor...Whoever gives to the poor lacks nothing...*(Proverbs 19:17, 22:9, 28:27).

Second, the staff did a wonderful thing by honoring her with this celebration. The results that come from wisdom are described in the following way: *"Esteem her (wisdom), and she will exalt you; embrace her, and she will honor you. She will set a garland of grace on your head and present you with a crown of splendor"* (Proverbs 4:8-9). When wisdom is used honor and splendor are given. That is what the staff was giving "See See." Let us keep serving whether we are ninety or thirty and wisdom will be setting a crown of splendor on our heads as well! Helping others is a motivation that brings blessings.

THE LOVE MOTIVATION PRESCRIPTION

When motivated he adheres to a weight loss and meal plan regimen. Trouble is most of the time he's not in the mood. When motivated he's driven to accomplish what he needs. Being motivated is the key, but not motivated in the sense of "in the mood", but rather the reason, purpose, the why for doing something. Imagine a person saying "I just can't exercise because I feel immediately tired and breathless, and my knees hurt when I've tried." So, there is no willpower or motivation. What if a wealthy benefactor offered him a thousand dollars to walk around the block, could he do it? Almost everyone could. What if each day the person was offered another hundred dollars to continue to walk while also adding additional steps each day? At the end of the week another thousand dollars is given. Also, the offer of one thousand is offered for each subsequent week of walking. As long as additional steps are added each week a thousand dollars awaits him. When he reaches 10,000 steps per day, a thousand dollars will be given each week to maintain the regimen. Is this achievable? Sure, the motivation for the money is there which in turn creates the willpower to accomplish it.

Will you ever receive an offer like that? I'm sure you can confidently say no! But do you know you actually have a better offer waiting for you today? Yes, today! And here it is—*"Blessed are those who find wisdom, those who gain understanding, for she is more profitable than silver and yields better returns than gold. She is more precious than rubies; nothing you desire can compare with her. Long life is in her right hand; in her left hand are riches and honor. Her ways are pleasant ways, and all her paths are peace. She is a tree of life to those who take hold of her; those who hold her fast will be blessed"* (Proverbs 3:13-18). Here is an offer of wisdom that is more precious than silver, gold or rubies. Now listen to what God or wisdom says—*"I love those who love me, and those who seek me find me"* (Proverbs 8:17). God gives his wisdom for us to use in this life because he loves us. His wisdom is for victory or success in life. *"For the LORD gives wisdom; from his mouth come knowledge and understanding. He holds success in store for the upright"* (Proverbs 2:6-7).

An example of how God's wisdom can motivate is found in this proverb—*"A friend loves at all times. He is there to help when trouble comes"* (Proverbs 17:17 NIrV). The following story illustrates this proverb. Two men in World War 1 who had been friends since childhood were on patrol one night. One has written, "That night while on patrol, our unit was ambushed. Shots rang out from all directions. Fortunately, most of us fell into the ditch that provided us with protection. Then, out in the darkness, I could hear my friend, Jim, calling for help. He kept calling my name. 'Gerry! Come and help me!' My captain ordered me to remain. He told me that there was no way I could save Jim and I would just get myself killed. But Jim kept calling me and I kept begging. Finally, he gave up and said, 'Okay! If you want to get yourself killed, go ahead.' I crawled across the ground in the darkness, got Jim and dragged him back to the ditch. After pushing him to safety, I fell into the ditch on top of him. It was then I realized that Jim was dead. The captain yelled at me. 'See! I told you there was no point to going out there.' But I told my captain that I had done the right thing. When I got to Jim, he was still alive. And the last thing he said to me was, 'Gerry, I knew you'd come.'" Yes, it is as the proverb says, *"A friend loves at all times."*

Their deep-seated friendship of love motivated Gerry to have the willpower to rescue his friend!

In the gratitude prescription mentioned in chapter one, looking on the brighter side of life, listing things for which we are thankful helps for willpower. People find it much easier to come up with a list of things for which they're thankful when they focus on blessings from others. Research on gratitude by Dr. Emmons at Cal-Davis University indicates this. So, how can we get things done especially for our health? [42] Focus on the little contributions you receive from others and can make for others. In other words, be kind and loving toward others. Use love as a motivation to get things done. Don't wait for someone to be kind to you. Be kind. Remember, God loves you! *"Do not forsake wisdom, and she will protect you; love her, and she will watch over you...do not let wisdom and understanding out of your sight, preserve sound judgment and discretion; they will be life for you, an ornament to grace your neck. Then you will go on your way in safety, and your foot will not stumble"* (Proverbs 4:6, 3:21-23).

INTRINSIC MOTIVATION PRESCRIPTION

Some people's motivation tank is empty. *"As a door turns on its hinges, so a sluggard turns on his bed"* (Proverbs 26:14). Notice what the person is called--a sluggard or good-for-nothing person. What if a sum of money was offered to get out of bed, would he? Maybe he would; maybe he wouldn't! Motivation that comes from outside a person like a reward or money is "extrinsic" motivation. When the money is gone, the motivation is gone. On the other hand, "intrinsic" motivation empowers a person within! Consider the following example.

At the beginning of the school year, an eighth-grade class of thirty-three students took a field trip. The principal noticed something unusual about them--they were surprisingly cooperative and having a good time. Physical fighting was the norm for handling conflicts among this class, but now they talk instead of fight. Why? They each will receive a reward of one hundred dollars at the end of the school year if none of them, yes none of them, get in a fight! If just one fights, no one will get the reward! The school is located in a poverty- stricken area of Philadelphia. Many of the students have food insecurity and have to live independently with rarely seen parents. The hundred-dollar reward was a great "extrinsic" motivation which transformed into "intrinsic" motivation. Their attitudes have changed; they now see better ways to resolve conflicts. No one wants to disappoint their classmates! Many are considered as role models; they know others look up to them.

The apostle Paul was one who had "intrinsic" motivation and he also had a *"thorn in the flesh."* The very word *"thorn"* indicates an intermittent almost unbearable pain. We don't know what this pain was, but the oldest of all theories is that Paul suffered from severe and prostrating headaches. He came into the Roman province of Galatia to teach. He wrote, *"As you know, it was because of an illness that I first preached the gospel to you"* (Galatians 4:13). He prayed three times that this *"thorn"* be taken from him, but God's answer was *"My grace is sufficient for you, for my power is made perfect in weakness"* (2 Corinthians 12:9). If he had the reward of no pain (extrinsic motivation), what would he have been able to accomplish? Instead, because of his gratitude for God's grace, gift or love, he was inwardly compelled to give exceptional service. *"Are they servants of Christ?... I am more. I have worked much harder, been in prison more frequently, been flogged more severely, and been exposed to death again and again...For Christ love compels us"* (2 Corinthians 11:23, 5:14). We see in him how "intrinsic" motivation empowers. For the students their motivation started with a hundred-dollar reward but turned into attitudes being changed to cooperate and become model students!

Watch: "School Marked By Violence Offers Cash Reward For Kids To Stop Fighting | NBC Nightly News" at https://www.youtube.com/watch?v=8n8mHpY2Wlg

CHAPTER FOUR

The Power of Movement

---

*"Go to the ant, you sluggard; consider its ways and be wise! It has no commander, no overseer or ruler, yet it **stores** its provisions in summer and **gathers** its food at harvest"* (Proverbs 6:6-8).

"Motivation" and "Purpose" are two important factors for success. Tom Hill was in the news for achieving fifty-two years and thirty-nine days. His age? No, these were consecutive days of running at least one mile per day.[43] At the age of seventy-eight he stopped only because his heart started hurting, becoming worse and worse during the last half of a one-mile run. He thought he'd better stop for his wife, family and friends. During the first fifty years he averaged seven miles a day. He isn't the only one running at least one mile every single day. According to Streak Runners International, thousands are. Jon Sutherland now has the record of consecutive days running, at forty-seven years and eight months. Watch "Runners go to crazy lengths for decades-long streaks" https://www.youtube.com/watch?v=CX85GdPmALw

Are they running to live or living to run? Once a man was asked why he was digging a ditch. "I've got to have money." "Why do you need money?" "To buy food." "Why do you need food?" "To have strength." "Why do you need strength?" "To dig ditches." His life was an endless cycle with no real purpose. "Streakers" may say they run to stay in good physical condition and/or because they enjoy it, but the motivating factor of maintaining a streak can take over! Why does a person run twenty days with painful injuries or run just the one-mile minimum required? Yes, many of these "streakers" do have a motivation—to keep their streak of consecutive days going.

What motivates us? Are we walking to live or living to walk? We know walking has physical benefits. So, why aren't more people walking? Lack of motivation? Does the following statement motivate you? *"For the LORD gives wisdom; from his mouth come knowledge and understanding. He holds success in store for the upright"* (Proverbs 2:7-8). Success is motivational; it helps us focus on a goal. And God gives his wisdom for us to succeed, to have victory in life. God cares about us! His wisdom blesses us! *"Blessed are those who find wisdom, those who gain understanding"* (Proverbs 3:13). So, from his wisdom he gives instructions for something as mundane as walking. *"Go to the ant...; consider its ways and be wise... it stores its provisions in summer and gathers its food at harvest"* (Proverbs 6:6-8). Ants move to store up their provisions. Likewise, if we are wise, we'll move too. God's wisdom helps and He blesses us when we use it! Let that motivate us! So, let's go to the scriptures, God's wisdom and be wise! Here are two more examples of that wisdom at work.

A recent news headline was "Houston hero rescues neighbors from Harvey's floodwaters." Video showed Howard Harris rescuing people from flood waters in his neighborhood in Cypress, Texas. After the last time his hometown flooded, he purchased a boat. He would be ready to evacuate neighbors safely if it happened again and that is what he was doing. Watch at https:// www.youtube.com/watch?v=jV34pjvYwyQ What a motivation! What difference can one man make? Ask his neighbors! This is just one of multiple stories of rescue during this storm!

A ninety-four-year-old woman jogged and walked a half-marathon race in San Diego with a similar motivation—to help people! When Harriette Thompson crossed the finish line, she made a goal for the second time. She became the oldest woman to ever finish the half-marathon, but two years before she was the oldest woman to complete a marathon.[44] Does she enter the marathons for the thrill of running? No, she runs to help others through funding cancer research. She has lost multiple family members, including in 2014 her husband of sixty-seven years, to cancer. She started raising funds in this way when she was seventy-six. Harriette has raised more than 115,000 dollars for research for the Leukemia & Lymphoma Society by running marathons. What a motivation! Helping those in need is God's wisdom at work. *"Blessed is the one who is kind to the needy"* (Proverbs 14:21). Watch "92-year-old woman breaks marathon record" at https://www.youtube.com/watch?v=cwL6BV_uKfs

Here are two more examples of getting exercise with a purpose—a man who walked 3,000 miles and a man walking fifteen miles a day to work. Then we'll examine the benefits of walking, the stand-up prescription and the 10,000 steps a day prescription.

NOT JUST WALKING 3,000 MILES

Walking along the southern border of the United States would be a daunting task for most people. This is a story of a ninety-year-old man who was determined to do it. He wasn't just ninety when he finished, he was ninety-three! Yes, it took him three years to reach his goal of the shores in Georgia. He started in San Diego on October 7, 2013, and thirty-four months later he reached his destination. How did he accomplish this? He would run five miles and then get a ride back to his vehicle. Two days later he would do the same thing, which is the nuts and bolts of what he did. How was Ernie Andrus, a World War II veteran, really inspired to do it? [45]

Motivation was how! He said, "I want people to know what the war was all about and what it took to win it." He specifically wanted people to know the kind of ship that made the difference for victory—LST (Landing Ship-Tank). These ships transported heavy equipment used in places like Normandy on D-Day. He was a medic on one of them. He knew of one—The Indiana—that could be renovated and used for the 75th anniversary of D-Day in France in 2019. That is why seventy years later he was running to give these ships the credit they deserve and collecting funds for the renovations. He said, "I'm running the whole thing, every step of the way." He started off walking by himself, but that didn't last long. When news spread about what this ninety-year-old veteran was doing, others started walking with him. He had up to 2,000 people following him in Louisiana.

Ernie had a real hunger to do this. Hunger or appetite drives a person on according to this proverb: *"The appetite of laborers works for them; their hunger drives them on"* (Proverbs 16:26). Willpower may be hard to come by. When there is a captivating purpose, a motivation, willpower naturally flows from it. It is what a person wants that propels a person to do what is necessary to fulfill a desire. The motivation in this proverb is to fulfill the need of hunger by working. A hunger, a need to be fulfilled, is a real purpose or motivation.

Nothing seemed to stop Ernie. He continued his walk for 3,000 miles, no matter the weather or how he may have felt. Let's have that kind of determination for our walk (or purpose in life) with no stopping for the roadblocks we may face. Let's consider a need or purpose that we have—to help others and give honor to God! *"Whoever is kind to the needy honors God...A generous person will prosper; whoever refreshes others will be refreshed...A good person gives life to others; the wise person teaches others how to live...Let your light shine before others, that they may see your good deeds and glorify your Father in heaven"* (Proverbs 14:31, 11:25, 11:30, Matthew 5:16).

Watch: "WWII vet runs 3,000 miles across the U.S."
https://www.youtube.com/watch?v=_GgJkQp_JBU

ONE STEP AT A TIME AND THEN SOME

A secretary of State from the 1930's James Francis Burns said, "I discovered at an early age that most of the differences between average people and great people can be explained in three words—and then some." What does "and then some" mean? Officer Branson found out. He said, "My kids will know about Patrick, my grandkids will know about Patrick, everyone should know about Patrick." Why did he want everyone to know about a man named Patrick? His characteristics of commitment, loyalty, perseverance, hard work, gratitude and integrity were the reasons. He was demonstrating the "and then some" principle. One day officer Branson saw this man walking along the side of the road. He pulled over and found out why.

Patrick had been transferred from one Braum's restaurant in Plano, Texas to another one in McKinney, Texas. The new one was about fifteen miles away from his home. When Patrick was interviewed about the position it was his opportunity for advancement in the company. When he was asked by Braum's management if he had reliable transportation he said he did.[46]

They didn't know his reliable transportation was his own two feet. His means of travel was brought to their attention from a post on the McKinney Police Department's Facebook page. Officer Branson posted Patrick's picture with himself on the Department's Facebook page with his story. In just twenty-four hours the post received more than 5000 likes and 1200 shares. Why would people have such an interest in such a post?

I've known people who have walked to their office. Sometimes the office is in their home. I don't know of anyone who would walk to work taking two and a half to three hours to get there. That is the "and then some" principle in action. He had been walking that distance for seven months when officer Branson talked with him. A friend would give him a ride home. When asked why he was doing it he said, "Commitment—you make a commitment to your job, to go to work every day. They expect you to go to work every day. No excuses." Patrick was also demonstrating God's way of wisdom. Proverbs 14:23 states, *"All hard work brings a profit, but mere talk leads only to poverty or "Work and you will earn a living; if you sit around talking you will be poor* (GNT)." He certainly wasn't just sitting around talking! He would work five days a week and then some—one step at a time for two and a half hours before he got there! *"The lazy will not get what they want, but those who work hard will"* (Proverbs 13:4 NCV).

STAND UP PRESCRIPTION

What does God's wisdom say about work? *"Those who work their land will have abundant food, but those who chase fantasies have no sense...From the fruit of their lips people are filled with good things, and the work of their hands brings them reward...All hard work brings a profit, but mere talk leads only to poverty"* (Proverbs 12:11,14, 14:23). Work brings monetary and material rewards, but the common work in 1000 BC, the time these proverbs were written, brought another type of reward. Here is an example of that type of work. *"Let me go to the fields and pick up the leftover grain behind anyone in whose eyes I find favor." Naomi said to her, "Go ahead, my daughter." So she went out, entered a field and began to glean behind the harvesters. As it turned out, she was working in a field belonging to Boaz* (Ruth 2:2-3). This type of work would bring monetary rewards, but this type of work would also bring another type of reward—physical health. Movement, lifting, turning, guiding a plow with an ox, harvesting a crop by hand would all be normal. Images like that would come to people's minds as they thought of these proverbs. Sitting in front of a desk would not enter the mind of the wise, but rather standing and moving jobs would—manual labor!

Recent books have been written with titles like "Sitting Kills, Moving Heals: How Everyday Movement Will Prevent Pain, Illness, and Early Death—and Exercise Alone Won't" by Joan Vernikos PhD or "Get Up!: Why Your Chair is Killing You and What You Can Do About It" by James Levine, MD. Dr. Vernikos was the Director of NASA's Life Sciences from 1993 to 2000 while Dr. Levine works for the Mayo Clinic. From the research discussed by both authors, too much sitting can be harmful to health. If we spend up to an hour exercising per day, what do we do the other twenty-three hours? Dr. Joan Vernikos recommends using gravity to our advantage. By just slowly standing up valuable changes take place in our body—changes like muscle contractions and nerve stimulations. One benefit of doing this is better blood pressure levels. The process of standing up is the stimulus, not the amount of time standing. The way to get the most benefit from standing up is to do it slowly and to stand up at least thirty-two times a day. "Stand up, sit less, move more" sums up research in avoiding sitting too much.

Standing has its own benefits. Dr. Francisco Lopez-Jimenez editorial on a research study of "Replacing sitting time with standing or stepping", summarizes the benefits of standing and stepping instead of sitting. The benefits are improved fasting blood glucose and triglyceride levels, a preventive to athero-genesis (formation of abnormal fatty or lipid masses in arte-rial walls). Also, by replacing standing with stepping results in better weight control.[47] If you work at a desk, a 20-8-2 ratio is recommended for every thirty minutes—that is sit for twenty minutes, stand for eight and move for two.[48]

10,000 STEPS OR MOVE MORE PRESCRIPTION

Should 10,000 steps per day be our goal? The way of wisdom instructs us to move more. *"Go to the ant, you sluggard; consider its ways and be wise!...Ants are creatures of little strength, yet they store up their food in the summer"* (Proverbs 30:25).

Just think of ants! What are some of their characteristics? They are fast and strong. Ants take the initiative. They don't let obstacles get in their way. They'll go over them, around them, or under them, which means they don't give up. They're per-sistent! They are always on the move—industrious, moving, saving, storing. In fact, how many couch potato ants have you seen? Of course, moving relates directly to our physical well-being and health.

So, should 10,000 steps per day be our goal? Who came up with the idea to walk 10,000 steps a day? In Japan, people were thinking about fitness about the time of the 1964 Tokyo Olympics. During that time, a Japanese company started sell-ing a pedometer called a "manpo-kei—"man" stands for 10,000, "po" for step and "kei" for gauge. It was a simple marketing campaign name by a Japanese company. The research behind the campaign was led by Doctor Yoshiro Hatano. He determined the average person took 3,500 to 5,000 steps per day and that if they were to increase their steps to 10,000 steps per day, the result should be healthier, thinner people!

Can we conclude that the Japanese diet of the 1960s was the same as the calorie rich diets of Americans today? For a few years, the number of Americans with diabetes and pre-diabetes was estimated at seventy-nine million people. The latest number released by the Centers for Disease Control and Prevention is one hundred fourteen million.[49] Are we today, as healthy as the Japanese were in the 1960s? Theodore Bestor, a Harvard researcher of Japanese society says that "By all accounts, life in Japan in the 1960s was less calorie-rich, less animal fat, and much less bound up in cars."[50] So, what should the number of steps per day be?

A study of Scottish postal workers found that the workers averaged 15,000 steps per day. And they were fit with normal waistlines, healthy cholesterol levels, and a lower risk of heart disease. What is the average number of steps of people per day in the United States? People in the U.S. only average 4,774 steps daily, according new Stanford University research.[51] Is this a healthy number? According to the CDC, obesity is present among more than one-third (36.5%) of U.S. adults, which also relates to this low number of daily steps.[52]

The Centers for Disease Control and Prevention recommends one hundred fifty minutes of moderate activity each week or 30 minutes of walking each day. They also recommend two days of muscle-strengthening activity.[53] How many total steps would you take if you walked the recommended 30-minute walk each day? Neil Johannsen, assistant Professor in the School of Kinesiology at Louisiana State University says some research indicates about 7,500 steps per day would be the total with a 30-minute walk included each day.

Sedentary people in the U.S. generally move only two to three thousand steps per day. Older adults and those living with chronic diseases typically take 3,500 to 5,500 steps per day. In one study, healthy older adults, who were sixty-nine years old and older, took about 6,600 steps per day, with almost 3,000 steps coming from structured, planned movement. This means they would have a structured walk of about one-and-a-half miles per day.[54]

Research indicates 10,000 steps or more per day is beneficial to health. One research study with hypertensive patients walking 10,000 steps per day resulted in lowering their blood pressure, increasing exercise capacity and reducing the sympathetic nerve activity. The sympathetic nervous system accelerates the heart rate, constricts blood vessels, and raises blood pressure. And this was not dependent on the intensity of the exercise or duration.[55] Another 10,000-step study of overweight women for four weeks improved blood glucose control and blood pressure even with no changes in body mass, body fat percentage, or waist circumference.[56]

So, would taking more steps each day be worth it? Of course, it would! First of all, find out what your average number of steps per day is by using a pedometer. After wearing a pedometer for a few days and finding your average number of steps per day, set your initial goal—6600, 7500 or 10000 or more steps per day. Put on your pedometer first thing in the morning and take it off right before going to bed. Start adding a few steps each day until you reach your goal. Adding a few steps each day is the best approach. The way of wisdom teaches the power of the little by little approach. *"Money that comes easily disappears quickly, but money that is gathered little by little will grow"* (Proverbs 13:11 NCV). Remember, *"For the LORD gives wisdom; from his mouth come knowledge and understanding. He holds success in store for the upright"* (Proverbs 2:6-7).

CHAPTER FIVE

The Power of Nutritious Eating

"A meal of vegetables where there is love is better than the finest meat where there is hatred" (Proverbs 15:17 NIrV).

E ating healthy is a challenge especially when there are so many delicious unhealthy temptations. People think that if they just practice some portion control they will succeed. Like Yogi Berra said, *"When the waitress asked if I wanted my pizza cut into four or eight slices, I said, 'Four. I don't think I can eat eight."*

Over the last twenty years serving sizes have drastically changed. A typical cheeseburger was 333 calories, today it is 590 calories. French fries were 210 calories and today a serving size is a whopping 610 calories. A soda was 85 calories and today a typical soda is 250 calories.[57] I'm not advocating eating those kinds of food but serving sizes for all foods has increased. A good idea to practice is to eat half of what is served at a restaurant and take the rest home.

People use fad diets to shed pounds quickly. Once the weight is shed the diet is dropped and old habits replace the diet with the weight lost being put back on and then some. Dr. Jennifer Hubert of St. Joseph Health Medical Group calls this yo-yo dieting. She says, "Other findings indicate that yo-yo dieting may lead to a higher risk of increased body fat, which means these diets, in the long run, can have the opposite of the intended effect of losing weight. What's worse is that most yo-yo dieting is done with the trendy diets of the moment, which are poor nutritionally compared to eating a regular diet of whole foods."[58]

"Our greatest weakness lies in giving up. The most certain way to succeed is always to try just one more time" said Thomas Edison. The way of wisdom states that *"A wise man has great power and a man of knowledge increases strength"* (Proverbs 24:5). The best way to do the "one more time" is with more knowledge. The following story tells of a woman winning a race at the age of one hundred. When I read her story, I was impressed with the insights she had for living.

WINNING THE RACE

Pleasantly surprising stories make for enjoyable reading. Consider this one about a woman winning the 100-yard dash at the 122nd Annual Penn Relays. To read about someone winning a race is not surprising, but to have someone competing and winning who is 100 years old is! Ida Keeling won while competing against many who were much younger, since she was in the eighty years and older category. She not only won, but also broke the world record for her age group!

Ida didn't start running until she was sixty-seven! A family tragedy motivated her daughter, Shelly Keeling, to enroll her in a 5K run. "She was just sitting at home in gloom." Shelly continues, "Both my brothers had been murdered, so she was sinking very quickly. I just picked her up one morning and said, 'you're coming with me,' and I bought her an extra pair of sneakers and the rest is history."

What is her secret to longevity? "Eat for nutrition, not for taste," she said. "Do what you need to do, not what you want to do, and make sure you exercise at least once every day." Her daughter is astonished at what her mother is able to still do at her age. Although she explains "It's like every year it feels longer than a year, and the amount of your ability that gets compromised can be a lot." Ida, however, is taking it all in stride, literally! But probably the most important thing she said seemed like an after-thought in the story. She said, "I thank God every day for my blessings."[59]

Notice how God's wisdom could be acknowledged in the lives of this mother and daughter. *"Trust in the LORD with all your heart and lean not on your own understanding; in all your ways acknowledge him, and he will make your paths straight"* (Proverbs 3:5). When she was becoming depressed, Shelly got her mother to start running! That's encouragement. What are its results? *"Those who are kind benefit themselves...whoever refreshes others will be refreshed"* (Proverbs 11:17, 25). When Ida told her secrets to longevity of eating for nutrition, doing what you need to do and exercising each day, she was giving wise insights. *"The prudent give thought to their steps"* (Proverbs 14:15). For Ida it was not just thoughtful decisions, but literal steps too. The final idea she expressed was "I thank God every day for my blessings." Blessings are like good news. What happens when we focus on the good news? *"Good news gives health to your body"* (Proverbs 15: 30). Through these examples we've seen the wisdom of kindness, thoughtfulness, nutrition, exercise and gratitude. We can practice those things, too, while acknowledging God's wisdom. When we do, God says He will make our paths straight!

COMFORT FOODS

Many people think that certain kinds of foods, commonly called "comfort foods," will sooth them. Popular "comfort foods" are potato chips, ice cream, cookies, candy, mashed potatoes, French fries, chocolate and other simple, often indulgent meals or snacks. Many have little nutritional value and are highly dense foods. In other words, there is no satiety or "feeling full" value to them and soon people are craving more.

LOW-DENSITY, LESS CONCENTRATED WITH CALORIES FOODS

"Choosing foods that are less concentrated with calories—meaning you get a larger portion size with a fewer number of calories—can help you lose weight and control your hunger."[60] The way of wisdom teaches, *"Be careful what you think, because your thoughts run your life"* (Proverbs 4:23 NCV). In this case, think volume of foods like vegetables, fruits, and lean meat. Eating more vegetables and fruits, which are mainly comprised of water with fiber and other nutrients will help provide a much longer full feeling than foods that have a high concentration of fat. Watch Dr. Barbara Rolls explains "Volumetrics" at https:// www.youtube.com/watch?v=Y-aM5sG7jlc

Foods are categorized by calorie density or high density/ low density at www.calorieking.com with asterisks. For example, strawberries are given four asterisks while the donut hole is given one asterisk. Foods with four asterisks would be the foods that are very low in calories per gram and the volume of food you eat is greater than high density foods. The fewer asterisks a food has the greater number of calories it has per gram.

WHAT CAN WE LEARN FROM DANIEL?

As a captive in Babylon during the reign of king Nebuchadnezzar (605–562 BC), Daniel and his three friends were being trained to be wise men in the royal courts. Their acclimation into the Babylonian culture included what they would eat and drink and was decided by the king. Daniel objected that the food would defile him spiritually, so he appealed to the officer to let them eat vegetables instead. The officer said, *"Why should he see you looking worse than the other young men your age?"* Daniel said to him, *"Please test your servants for ten days: Give us nothing but vegetables to eat and water to drink. Then compare our appearance with that of the young men who eat the royal food, and treat your servants in accordance with what you see"* (Daniel 1:10,12-13). What happened?

"So he agreed to this and tested them for ten days. At the end of the ten days they looked healthier and better nourished than any of the young men who ate the royal food" (Daniel 1:14–15). What they were eating were water, nutrient-rich foods that come in fruits and vegetables. In other words, they were eating whole

foods. It worked 2,700 years ago for health and wellness, and it will still work today!

WHOLE FOODS

Whole foods are like the difference between an apple and apple juice. The way to have fruit is in its whole state with all the nutrients still there. Plus, in the whole state foods are much more filling! Healthy whole foods naturally are loaded with fiber, vitamins and minerals. Some are antioxidants. Antioxidants protect cells against damage. Whole foods are the state of rich nutrient-dense foods. They have little or no added sugars, fats and exclude added salt or other ingredients high in sodium. Some of the most nutrient rich foods are turnip and mustard greens, kale, spinach, brussel sprouts, radishes, cabbage, red peppers, romaine lettuce, tomatoes, cauliflower, strawberries, blackberries, raspberries, blueberries, oranges, apples, beans (not canned) and walnuts.[61] Other nutrient-dense foods include whole grains, seafood, eggs, peas, unsalted nuts and seeds, fat-free and low-fat dairy products, and lean meats and poultry.62

A PROVERB ABOUT A MEAL OF VEGETABLES

Remember that the basic meaning of the word proverb is represent, compare or be like. Proverbs give pictures of life. Notice how the picture of love and hatred is contrasted and portrayed in the following Proverb: *"A meal of vegetables where there is love is better than the finest meat where there is hatred"* (Proverbs 15:17 NIrV). Most people find a meal of delicious steak very satisfying to the taste, but the taste is lost when eating the meal with those who are bitter, resentful and hateful toward you.

Whereas, the picture of a meal with those you love is pictured with vegetables. And guess what? As we've been examining, vegetables are good for us. Isn't it interesting that a subtle message of a meal with love is portrayed with vegetables, which are very beneficial to good health!

EAT FIBER RICH FOODS

On food labels, fiber is counted in the total number of carbohydrate grams. Fiber, however, is actually a complex carbohydrate that the body can't break down. It has several benefits such as helping to prevent blood glucose spikes after a meal, control food cravings, give a longer lasting full feeling and helps with weight control since more volume of food is eaten with less calories. So, how much fiber do we need in order to reap the benefits? According to the American Dietetic Association twenty to thirty-five grams are recommended per day, and of that, 5—10 grams should be soluble fiber. Americans only get about 15 or less grams of total fiber per day. Drink plenty of water per day (34-64 ounces) because fiber works best when it absorbs water.[63]

There are two types of fiber: insoluble and soluble. Insoluble fiber absorbs water, but does not dissolve in it. Insoluble fiber is found in such foods as bran flakes, bran muffins and whole wheat bread. Soluble fiber dissolves in water and becomes a gummy gel, which slows down the absorption of glucose and helps blunt elevated blood glucose after a meal. Soluble fiber is found in such foods as apples, citric fruits, oat bran, oatmeal, dried beans and peas.[64] For example, Bob's Red Mill™ Oat Bran cereal has 7 grams of fiber per serving of which 2 grams is soluble fiber. Bob's Red Mill™ Rolled Oats cereal has 5 grams of fiber per serving which includes 1.6 grams soluble fiber.

From information supplied by Harvard University Health Services, I've selected a list of foods which are especially rich in soluble fiber and should be included in our meal plans.[65]**Each food is listed with serving size, then total fiber grams per serving and the number of grams of soluble fiber included in each serving.**

Cooked Vegetables:
- Asparagus ½ cup 2.8, 1.7
- Broccoli ½ cup 2.4, 1.2
- Brussels sprouts ½ cup 3.8, 2.0
- Carrots, sliced ½ cup 2.0, 1.1
- Okra, frozen ½ cup 4.1, 1.0
- Peas, green, frozen ½ cup 4.3, 1.3
- Sweet Potato, flesh only ½ cup 4.0, 1.8
- Turnip ½ cup 4.8, 1.7

Raw Vegetables:
- Carrots, fresh 1, 7 ½ in. long 2.3, 1.1
- Celery, fresh 1 cup chopped 1.7, 0.7
- Onion, fresh ½ cup chopped 1.7, 0.9
- Pepper, green, fresh 1 cup chopped 1.7, 0.7

Fruits:
- Apple, red, fresh w/skin 1 small 2.8, 1.0
- Apricots, dried 7 halves 2.0, 1.1
- Apricots, 4 fresh w/skin 3.5, 1.8

- Figs, dried 1 ½ 3.0, 1.4
- Grapefruit, fresh ½ medium 1.6, 1.1
- Kiwifruit, fresh, flesh only 1 large 1.7, 0.7
- Orange, fresh, flesh only 1 small 2.9, 1.8
- Peach, fresh, w/skin 1 medium 2.0, 1.0 Pear, fresh, w/ skin ½ large 2.9, 1.1
- Plum, red, fresh 2 medium 2.4, 1.1
- Prunes, dried 3 medium 1.7, 1.0
- Raspberries, fresh 1 cup 3.3, 0.9
- Strawberries, fresh 1 ¼ cup 2.8, 1.1

Legumes (cooked):
- Black beans ½ cup 6.1, 2.4
- Black-eyed peas ½ cup 4.7, 0.5
- Chick peas, dried ½ cup 4.3, 1.3
- Kidney beans, light red ½ cup 7.9, 2.0
- Lentils ½ cup 5.2, 0.6
- Lima beans ½ cup 4.3, 1.1
- Navy beans ½ cup 6.5, 2.2
- Pinto beans ½ cup 6.1, 1.4

Breads and Crackers:
- Pumpernickel 1 slice 2.7, 1.2
- Rye 1 slice 1.8, 0.8

THE WISDOM WAY

"Be sure you know the condition of your flocks, give careful attention to your herds" (Proverbs 27:23). The principle of this wisdom teaching is to know the condition of what you own, which would include your own health. In other words, it is a good idea to keep track of what you eat. It is also appropriate to give thought to what you do, which would include what you eat and what exercise you get. *"The wisdom of the prudent is to give thought to their ways"* (Proverbs 14:8). *"The simple believe anything, but the prudent give thought to their steps"* (Proverbs 14:15). Wisdom also teaches about how much you eat, self-control and portion control when eating. *"The best food and olive oil are stored up in the houses of wise people. But a foolish man eats up everything he has"* (Proverbs 21:20 NIrV).

KEEP LEARNING PRESCRIPTION

"Intelligent people are always eager and ready to learn" (Proverbs 18:15).

Many people use the drive-thru window at McDonald's to place an order for cheeseburgers or chicken nuggets. Sometimes it saves time. Workers see a variety of cars, pickup trucks and vans. The ages of people vary as well. Recently workers saw a very unusual sight. A van pulled up, which wasn't unusual, but who was driving it was—an eight-year-old boy. Workers thought the parents were pulling a prank, thinking they were seated in the back seat, but to their surprise the only person in the back seat was the boy's four-year-old sister.

What would you do if you saw an eight-year-old driving a van? Witnesses saw him safely driving and called the police. He knew how to drive. In his mile-and-a-half trek from home he made several right turns and one left turn. He waited at traffic lights, drove over a railroad track, kept under the speed limit, and waited for traffic to pass before making his left turn. Then he drove up to McDonald's and placed his order.

When the policeman arrived, he didn't place any charges. He even allowed the siblings to eat their cheeseburgers. Grandparents were informed to pick them up by a customer who recognized the children. This all happened on a Sunday evening about 8 p.m. The boy had a hunger pang for a cheeseburger and didn't want to disturb his parents who were sleeping.

The boy said he had learned to drive by watching a YouTube video. "I think there is a good teaching point here. With the way technology is any more kids will learn how to do anything and everything," said the officer. "This kid learned how to drive on YouTube. He probably looked it up for five minutes and then said it was time to go."

Isn't it amazing what people, even an eight-year-old, can learn? According to the way of God's wisdom, knowledge empowers a person. *"A wise man has great power, and a man of knowledge increases strength"* (Proverbs 24:5). If more people had an attitude to learn like he did, it would make a difference in their lives. Of course, learning includes the wisdom of how and when to apply the knowledge. The learning attitude is needed no matter our age. The attitude is expressed in the following passage: *"Listen, my sons, to a father's instruction; pay attention and gain understanding. I give you sound learning, so do not forsake my teaching. For I too was a son to my father, still tender, and cherished by my mother. Then he taught me, and he said to me, "Take hold of my words with all your heart; keep my commands, and you will live. Get wisdom, get understanding; do not forget my words or turn away from them"* (Proverbs 4:1-5). God's wisdom will enable us to do things we otherwise couldn't do! Let's keep learning.

Watch: "Ohio 8-Year-Old Boy STEALS Father's Car and DRIVES Little Sister To McDonald's For CHEESEBURGERS!!" at https://www.youtube.com/watch?v=fJZkqwwBMXs

Keep learning about the foods that have nutritional value and eat them. Here is a starting list for all of us to consider. Potassium is a mineral and electrolyte that is found in potatoes, sweet potatoes, bananas, grape fruit, broccoli, avocados, salmon, grass-fed beef, peas and legumes. Potassium contributes to good blood pressure, heartbeat rhythms and nerve impulses. It contributes to digestive health and boosts energy levels.

"Magnesium plays a central role in just about every bodily process, from the synthesis of DNA to the metabolism of insulin" says Rachael Link, MS, RD. Often people with stomach or intestinal problems, type 2 diabetes, or just being an older adult have a deficiency in magnesium. Magnesium is a mineral and is found in such foods as spinach, dark chocolate, pumpkin seeds, almonds, black beans, avocado, dried figs, yogurt, and bananas. For more information on potassium, magnesium, calcium, vitamin A, C, and D, as well as an in-depth resource on nutritious food, educational videos and recipes go to Dr. Josh Axe Food is

Medicine website at https://draxe.com/ Read "Food Is Medicine: The Diet of Medicinal Foods, Science & History" at https://draxe.com/food-is-medicine/

FEEL FULL ON LESS CALORIES PRESCRIPTION

Eating foods that make you feel full have a high percentage of water content. Notice the water content of the following foods: fruits and vegetables (80–95%), hot cereal (85%), low-fat fruit-flavored yogurt (75%), boiled egg (75%), and fish and seafood (60–85%). When we compare a popular junk food like potato chips, we discover it has only 2 percent water content.[66]Researchers at Penn State University conducted a clinical trial for one year with seventy-one obese women age twenty-two to sixty. They wanted to determine if eating low-calorie, dense foods would facilitate the loss of weight as well as control hunger. They were assigned to one of two groups, each with different meal plan emphases. One was a meal plan with reduced fat content. The other group also had a reduced fat content, plus they were to eat foods high in water content. Neither group was given a daily calorie limit. People with diabetes, however, need to keep track of how many carbohydrates are eaten, because carbs affect blood glucose control. For more information on this read chapter eight through ten on 17 Wise Ways to Outsmart Diabetes on Daily Basis.

Weight was lost by both groups of women. The group that added more low-density calorie foods, the water-rich foods, ate 25 percent more food by weight, not calories; felt less hungry; and lost more weight. After six months, those on the meal plan of reduced fat lost 14.7 pounds, whereas the other group lost

19.6 pounds. "We have now shown that choosing foods that are low in calorie density helps in losing weight, without the restrictive messages of other weight loss diets," explained Dr. Julia A. Ello-Martin.[67]PLANNING AHEAD PRESCRIPTION BANK ATM: AN ODD WITHDRAWAL

Have you ever wished you had the opportunity to go back and do something differently? It might have involved words, or money, or time. For example, a man angry with his father decided to write him a scathing letter. He told a friend at work of the situation and he wrote his critical, bitter letter, telling his father to stay out of his business! His friend agreed to take his letter to the mailroom along with some others. (This was long before there was texting or email.) The next day he said, "I would give you a hundred dollars if I could have that letter back" for he regretted what he had done. It's been said "Speak when you are angry and you will make the best speech you'll ever regret." The friend then pulled out the letter from his pocket for he knew there might be second thoughts.

The desire to go back and do things differently happens in many situations. For example, have you ever locked your car and then looked in to see your keys sitting on the seat? Even worse, what if you got locked into an ATM service room? A recent news headline was "Texas Police Make Odd Withdrawal from ATM: A Man Who Was Trapped Inside." A contractor, who was changing the lock on the service room of an ATM, realized he had locked himself in the room. Plus, he couldn't call anyone for help because he had left his cell phone in his truck.[68]

What was he to do? He became very creative. People started receiving more than cash and a receipt at the ATM. They also got a handwritten note with their receipt—"Please Help. I'm stuck in here, and I don't have my phone. Please call my boss. At 210…" He did this for about two hours until one person finally took the message and called the police. "This is just a prank" is what most people thought, including the police until someone behind the screen answered them. They broke the door down and freed the desperate man. A police officer said, "We have a once-in-a-lifetime situation that you'll probably never see or hear about again."

What lessons can we learn from this? Ask for help when needed, or even better plan ahead. The way of God's wisdom teaches the importance of planning ahead, of not getting in a hurry, of not having the desire to go back and do things differently. *"The plans of the diligent lead to profit as surely as haste leads to poverty"* (Proverbs 21:5). *"Enthusiasm without knowledge is not good. If you act too quickly, you might make a mistake"* (Proverbs 19:2). We all need to plan ahead, and to think before doing!

Watch: "Police Withdraw Man Trapped In Bank ATM" at https://www.youtube.com/watch?v=ww81-eiwyzM

So, the following prescription is a plan that involves salads. Put it into your plans!

EATING A SALAD BEFORE THE MAIN COURSE PRESCRIPTION

What would happen if you ate a salad before each meal? Could the salad decrease the amount of food you eat for the entire meal? Forty-two women participated in a study conducted by the Department of Nutritional Sciences of Penn State University to research that very idea. Several lunch options were given for each lunch. The control condition was to not eat a salad before the main course of the meal, which was pasta. They were to eat as much pasta as they desired. The number of calories was measured.

Other lunch options were various sizes and energy densities of salads. The participants were required to eat the salads before the main course. The portion size of the salads used was either 150 grams or 300 grams by weight. The volume of salad on a plate was reduced by changing the amount and type of dressing and cheese. Obviously, the salad ended up being smaller when more dressing or cheese was used, bringing the weight to either 150 grams or 300 grams, but with less lettuce or vegetables. For example, the 150-gram salad came with three levels of total calories: fifty, one hundred, or two hundred calories. If it was the low-energy-density salad, it would be equal to about three cups of salad with a very light dressing. The 300-gram salad came with the same calculations (0.33, 0.67, or 1.33 kcal/g, or one hundred, two hundred, or four hundred total calories).[69]

According to this study, if you want to control weight or lose weight, eat a salad without high-calorie dressings or cheese before your main course at dinner or supper. The salads that pack more volume of food on the plate or in the bowl, but with fewer calories, resulted in less food eaten during the main course of pasta. In other words, starting a meal with this type of salad enhances satiety or the feeling of being full and thus reduces the amount of food eaten during the main course.

The study further determined that a salad for weight loss is an effective strategy when a large portion is eaten before meals. For the smaller salad of 150 grams, with a low-calorie dressing, 7 percent less was eaten for the main course; and for the 300-gram salad, it was 12 percent.

According to the research, if you use calorie-rich dressing like blue cheese, which has seventy-six calories and 8 grams of fat per serving, or Thousand Island dressing, which has sixty calories and almost 6 grams of fat, you will end up eating more for the main course. When two salads with the same number of calories were compared, it was found that meal intake was decreased when the large portion of the lower-energy-density salad was consumed; and meal intake was increased with the smaller portion of energy-dense salad that had weighty calorie laden salad dressing.

The message is clear—leave off the rich dressings! Use low-calorie dressings. Use dressings like vinaigrette or the wide assortment of Walden Farms no calorie dressings—https://www.waldenfarms.com/—and have more salad! One person in our diabetes support group began concentrating on eating more salad with the Walden Farms dressings. Tremendous benefits for her blood glucose levels resulted, going from an A1c of 12.4 (309 BG average) to an 8.2 A1c (189 BG average). Eat more salad and use nutrient rich Romaine lettuce!

One cup of romaine lettuce has 8 calories, 5 grams of fiber, vitamin A, K, C, iron, folate, manganese and potassium. It has high levels of antioxidants—vitamins mentioned above. The vitamin A is a deterrent to inflammation. We often cut the leaves and make a delicious salad.[70]

CHAPTER SIX

The Power of Stress Control

---

*"Peace of mind means a healthy body, but jealousy
will rot your bones."* (Proverbs 14:30 NCV).

You're driving along at the designated speed limit, enjoying the afternoon. You've just put your new up-to-date license tags on the car and all of a sudden you notice in your rear-view mirror flashing lights. You wonder what have I done now? Your heart is pounding, you're trembling and your throat is dry. As the officer approaches your pulse picks up, you're now sweating and you feel a tension headache starting! Once he gets to your car door he does something totally unexpected, in fact, shocking. He then compliments you for your good driving habits and gives you a gift card for a popular restaurant. He lets you know the police department has partnered with local restaurants to let the community know they appreciate law abiding citizens. Now you feel a sense of calm and peace.

Sometimes circumstances present themselves where a person doesn't even feel stressed, but an elevated blood glucose check reveals the presence of stress. After all factors are eliminated stress is the answer in certain situations. There are other times when one obviously feels stress like the example of the officer above. Some of the symptoms of acute stress are pounding heart, rapid pulse, trembling, shaky, dry throat and mouth, change in blood sugar level, sweating, diarrhea or frequent urination, indigestion and tension headache. Some of the signs and symptoms of chronic stress are general irritability, easily fatigued, depression, loss of appetite, anxiety, nervousness, chronic muscle pains and insomnia.[71]

Stress is an ever-present part of life, but we need to keep it under control. Stress often occurs at the doctor's office when your blood pressure it checked. White coat hypertension occurs because of anxiety in the situation resulting in an elevated blood pressure reading. A few minutes later when the blood pressure is checked the reading is lower because of less anxiety. When we perceive something as a threat or as stressful, like a conflict with someone, the brain recognizes the danger and releases an array of stress hormones like cortisol, epinephrine (adrenaline), and norepinephrine.[72]

I had a stressful experience at Silver Dollar City when I rode the "Giant Barn Swing." Weak was how I felt two hours after eating lunch. So before getting on the swing, I checked my blood glucose. My feelings were wrong. I was 162 mg/dl. Since I wasn't weak, I rode the swing with my family. After the two-minute ride I still felt weak. This time it was 197 mg/dl. My rapid increase in blood glucose was a result of stress! With elevated levels of the stress hormone cortisol, insulin is less effective. Thus, the result is higher blood glucose levels. To see what I experienced watch the "Giant Barn Swing at Silver Dollar City" at https://www.youtube.com/watch?v=irXWWIrKXwk

How can the way of wisdom help in stressful situations? When wisdom's way is followed, a more peaceful, composed lifestyle can result. *"My child, do not forget my teaching, but let your heart keep my commandments; for length of days and years of life and abundant welfare they will give you"* (Proverbs 3:1–2 NRS). Another Bible translation puts it the following way: *"My son, do not forget my teaching, but keep my commands in your heart, for they will prolong your life many years and bring you peace and prosperity."*

Several benefits stand out in this reading: a longer life, peace, and abundant welfare. In this case, the word *peace* can mean completeness or wholeness, and *prosperity* can mean abundant welfare. When a person puts this wisdom into practice, like the father instructs his son to do, then peace and abundant welfare can result. This peace will be with God, a calming peace within oneself, and in relationships with others. Conflict with others contributes to stress, which can directly affect blood glucose control and, thus, the management of diabetes!

Read the following two examples of stress. The first one demonstrates the importance of communication and the second one emphasizes choosing to avoid stressful situations. Then the following six prescriptions for coping with stress are given: taking life one day at a time, praying, bringing cheer to others, forgiving, staying hydrated with water and napping to avoid sleep deprivation.

COMMUNICATION

"As a tree gives fruit, healing words give life" (Proverbs 15:4).

Communication at times is very challenging and stressful. After all, "The difference between the almost right word and the right word is really a large matter—'tis the difference between the lightning bug and the lightning," wrote Mark Twain. The right words come with great difficulty sometimes like when two friends see each other for the first time in years. After their initial greetings one friend asked the other about his wife. "How's Martha doing?" He said, "She's no longer with me; she's in heaven." The man couldn't think of anything to say except "I'm sorry." Realizing that wasn't the best answer he changed it to "I'm glad." That still didn't have a good ring to it so in frustration he finally said, "Well, I'm surprised."

Yes, getting the right message across can be tough. This happened to two Tulsa police officers, Adam Ashley and Tempest Thorpe. They responded to a call to two young boys' house. "We realized they were deaf, we also realized they were Spanish-speaking deaf only," Ashley said. How to communicate with the family, who were all deaf, was the challenge. The Google Translator app solved the problem. "Hey, you can type in Spanish and I'll still understand. I just copy and paste into Google translator and problem solved," she said. They noticed the boys playing with fishing reels. When asked where their rods were, they said, "We don't have enough money for rods." That is when they decided to bring rods the next day and gave a pantomimed casting lesson.

The translator app accomplished the language problem, but much more was communicated than words. An act of kindness didn't need any translation! The boys understood the message of encouragement they received! The way of wisdom teaches the importance of using the right words, not the almost right words. *"A word fitly spoken is like apples of gold in a setting of silver"* (Proverbs 25:11). *"A person finds joy in giving an apt reply—and how good is a timely word!"* (Proverbs 15:23). *"The wise in heart are called discerning, and gracious* (pleasant) *words promote instruction"* (Proverbs 16: 21). People also understand the message of kind acts. *"Whoever is kind to the poor lends to the LORD, and he will reward them for what they have done"* (Proverbs 19:17).

If we really desire to say the right word in a fitting, pleasant way, consider the following:

Instead of: "You've got a long, hard road ahead of you." **Try:** "No matter what happens, I want you to know you're not alone."

Instead of: "My uncle had the same thing, and he died." **Try:** "What's going on with you today?"

Instead of: "I'm sure God has a reason for this." **Try:** There's a lot in life we don't understand, isn't there?"[73]

What we all need is the communication of pleasant, understanding words and kind acts!

AVOID STRESSFUL SITUATIONS: DRAMA IN THE SKY

A dramatic event took place in the skies of Australia when a skydiving student had a seizure 9,000-feet above ground. After jumping at 12,000 feet he went into a seizure after traveling about 3,000 feet. He then began a free fall, flipping over and going unconscious for about thirty seconds. His flight instructor was above him. He could see that something was wrong. With his diving skills he dove to catch up with the unconscious student pulling his ripcord. He regained consciousness at 3,000 feet above ground and made an uneventful landing. He had been the perfect student until this last terrifying jump. "I remember up until the point I blacked out and then waking up underneath the parachute at about 3,000 feet. I think I'm fairly lucky, but the emergencies [automatic activation devices] on the chutes work nearly all the time so I think I would have been OK if the jump master hadn't actually caught me."

The jump instructor knew Mr. Jones' parachute would automatically deploy, but "given the circumstances" he wanted to help. "At no time was I worried he was going to hit the ground without a parachute, but given the circumstances and where we were I thought it would be better to get him under parachute earlier than later," Mr. McFarlane said. "I managed to catch him on my second attempt and deploy his parachute. "As far as difficult, yeah, it was OK. I got him." "We don't do it all day every day, but part of our training is to look after students." Jones' video of the Nov. 14 incident, which he posted Sunday (3.3.15), already has more than 4 and a half million views at YouTube. (As of 5/22/18 it has 18 and a half million views) "GUY HAS

SEIZURE WHILE SKYDIVING" https://www.youtube.com/watch?v=55QUQHm2B5A

What lessons from God's wisdom can we learn from this incident? I see at least three ways God's wisdom, the skill for living can be applied. Are we using the proper equipment? First, Proverbs 14:4 states *"Where there are no oxen, the manger is empty, but from the strength of an ox comes an abundant harvest."* In ancient times oxen were essential equipment for major agricultural endeavors (read Deut. 22:1,10; 25:4). A broader meaning of this proverb is that we must obtain and use the right equipment to get the best results. The best equipment for us, in a sense, is God's wisdom. Proverbs 4:11-13 states that it keeps us from stumbling in life. Second, Proverbs 14:8 states *"The wisdom of the prudent is to give thought to their ways, but the folly of fools is deception."* Was the student giving full thought to his ways by taking these classes? He will not be taking any more classes because the stress of jumping triggered the episode. We need to give thought to all of our decisions as well! Avoid unnecessary stressful situations. Third, Proverbs 14:21 states *"It is a sin to despise one's neighbor, but blessed are those who are kind to the needy."* The flight instructor saw someone in need and helped him. When we see someone in need, let's do the same!

ONE DAY AT A TIME PRESCRIPTION

Peace at all times? Yes, all times according to 2 Thessalonians 3:16. *"Now may the Lord of peace himself give you peace at all times and in every way. The Lord be with all of you."* How can we have peace at all times? We know that worry is a great obstacle to peace. It is not uncommon for people to put off living in the present in order to worry about the future, or to yearn for some "magical rose garden over the horizon." And yet Jesus instructs us to live one day at a day, doing the best we can each day. He gives the following instruction to the disciples on how to pray: *"Give us today our daily bread"* (Matthew 6:11). Living one day at a time, breaking our lives into smaller compartments, makes a difference in overcoming worry!

When Thomas Carlyle had finished writing his history of the French Revolution, he took the manuscript to a neighbor, John Stuart Mill, for proofreading. A few days later, Mill came to Carlyle's house with disastrous news. His maid had used the manuscript to start a fire in the fireplace. Carlyle raged like a madman for several days. For two whole years he had poured himself into writing that manuscript. Now two years of his life were reduced to ashes. Carlyle thought he could never again give himself to the difficult discipline of writing.

One day he stood looking out his second story window where across the way he saw a stone mason slowly and patiently rebuilding a collapsed wall. "It came to me," he wrote later, "that as they lay brick on brick, so could I still lay word on word, sentence on sentence." And he did! This is how Jesus teaches us to live life--one day at a time. He says, *"Therefore, do not worry about tomorrow for tomorrow will worry about itself. Each day has enough trouble of its own"* (Matthew 6:34). Laying one day on another is the way to live, have peace and win over worry and stress!

PRAYER PRESCRIPTION

God's wisdom can be used anywhere and at any age. Even at a Waffle House? Yes, even at a Waffle House! "5-Year-Old Alabama Boy's Act of Kindness Moves Homeless Man, Restaurant Patrons to Tears" was a positive headline.[74] Obviously, the any age is five. The boy and his mother were at a Waffle House one evening when in walked a homeless man. His appearance grabbed the boy's attention. He started peppering his mom with many questions. She thought he was homeless. He asked, "What is that?" She explained that he didn't have a house where he could sleep and live. When he understood what that meant he insisted that his mother buy him a meal. So that is exactly what she did. Then her son wanted to take the meal to the man. It was when he took the meal to the man that the eleven people in the restaurant were touched, bringing some to tears. Before the man could take his first bite, Josiah, the five-year old insisted on saying a prayer. And he did it loud enough for everyone to hear. "The man cried. I cried. Everybody cried," said his mother, Ava.

"Watching my son touch the eleven people in that Waffle House tonight will be forever one of the greatest accomplishments as a parent I'll ever get to witness," Ava wrote. "You never know who the angel on Earth is, and when the opportunity comes you should never walk away from it," she added. I think she was referring to a passage in Hebrews. *"Do not forget to show hospitality to strangers, for by so doing some people have shown hospitality to angels without knowing it"* (Hebrews 13:2). We too can touch others by praying for them. Prayer will help us too.

According to God's wisdom, pleasant words bring healing to the body. *"Pleasant words are like honey. They are sweet to the spirit and bring healing to the body"* (Proverbs 16:24 NIrV). Sometimes we don't know what to say or how to pray. Then let's try praying with the apostle Paul.

"May you be made strong with all the strength that comes from his glorious power, and may you be prepared to endure everything with patience, while joyfully giving thanks to the Father" (Colossians 1:11-12 NRS).

The very words of that prayer are pleasant. They are words from God! When we pray that prayer of pleasant words, God is already giving hope in facing difficult stressful challenges, including concerns with our health. We will prosper!

When we hear about others taking our name to the creator of the universe, we are encouraged! From a scientific research standpoint praying for others has been found to be therapeutic. Thousands were interviewed for research done at the University of Michigan.[75] Interviews were conducted to see if praying for others could reduce the effects of financial strain on the health and well-being of those praying. The conclusion was that praying does reduce financial stress and improve health. Many people pray for things like new cars, better houses, and money. No benefits for health or protection from the effects of financial stress resulted with an inward focus. Praying for others was the key for better health. Focus on praying for others! Let them know. That was the approach of the Apostle Paul! Praying for others can be done anywhere, even at a Waffle House.

CHEERFUL HEART IS GOOD MEDICINE
PRESCRIPTION: "GOOD NIGHT" LIGHTS

"A cheerful heart is good medicine, but a crushed spirit dries up the bones" (Proverbs 17:22). While bearing a crushed, discouraging attitude it is difficult to do anything. Good medicine, as a cheerful heart, can prevent a crushed attitude! That kind of medicine is needed especially for youth confined in children's hospitals, facing numerous ailments including cancer.

The very fact that a child is confined in a hospital would be stressful. Add to that the painful procedures would make the stay very difficult. In children's hospitals distractions (like story books or music boxes) are used to divert children's attention away from painful procedures. They help them focus on pleasant thoughts and special places. The way of wisdom states *"Pleasant words are like honey. They are sweet to the spirit and bring healing to the body"* and *"Be careful what you think, because your thoughts run your life"* (Proverbs 16:24 NIrV, 4:23 NCV).

The Hasbro Children's Hospital in Providence, RI, found an innovative way to give doses of cheerful heart medicine. They use "Good Night" lights. A volunteer cartoonist started this practice in 2010. He would usually ride his bike home each night, but one night he stopped about a quarter of a mile away, focused on a teenager's room, and flashed his bike lights toward the window. The boy, who would be dismissed the next day, flickered his room lights in return. They were exchanging a message of "good night" with their lights. From that night on this "Good Night" lights routine started.

Now at 8:30 each evening the children gather near windows to see flickering lights and they flicker their flashlights in return.

Steve Brosnihan, the volunteer cartoonist, began asking others to participate. Now restaurants, police with their patrol lights, an assisted living center, and people from the community participate. They send their lights signifying "good night" and the children return a "thank you" with their lights. Wisdom teaches that *"Whoever seeks good finds favor or goodwill"* (Proverbs 11:27). This is precisely what the children are finding—goodwill. This is bringing stress-relief not only to them but to those giving the goodwill to them! *"Whoever refreshes others will be refreshed"* (Proverbs 11:25).

A toddler, after brain surgery, is thrilled with this activity each evening. A 13-year-old girl, after getting out of 5-day stay in a windowless intensive care unit, is excited to see the lights for the first time and is grateful that strangers take the time to do this. Her mom thinks the activity is genius because it lifts the children's spirits without any cost. The assisted living residents feel they are contributing to making children's lives better. This is good news! God's wisdom says, *"A cheerful look brings joy to your heart. And good news gives health to your body"* (Proverbs 15:30). These children receive cheerful, flickering lights bringing joy to their difficult lives. Let's think of ways we, too, can give cheer to others because it is good medicine! *"Let your light shine before others, that they may see your good deeds and glorify your Father in heaven"* (Matthew 5:16).

Watch: "How the City Of Providence Comforts Sick Children | NBC Nightly News" https://www.youtube.com/watch?v=D1HAWGZPfCU

Watch: "Good Night Lights tradition spans river, generations" https://www.youtube.com/watch?v=o3Wg2OWRGqU

FORGIVENESS PRESCRIPTION

Jesus' teachings apply to life. Practice his teachings; they are so relevant to truly living. This was vividly displayed recently by a man in the news. The teaching he demonstrated is this—*"For if you forgive other people when they sin against you, your heavenly Father will also forgive you. But if you do not forgive others their sins, your Father will not forgive your sins"* (Matthew 6:14-15). If we say, "I will never forgive so-and-so for what he or she did to me" or "I will never forget what so-and-so did to me" then can we pray this prayer? Are we deliberately asking God to not forgive us? Is that what Jesus means?

The headline read "Wrongfully Convicted Man Holds No Grudge after Spending 24 Years in Prison."[76] Shaurn was convicted of a crime when he was only nineteen. He was sentenced for life. Evidence was found after almost two-and-a-half decades that acquitted, or cleared, him of guilt in the case. He was released, said he felt wonderful, and couldn't feel better! The first thing he wanted to do was go to Red Lobster and have the "Ultimate Feast." As he sat there with his friends, he used a cell phone for the first time. When asked about being wrongfully convicted, he gave some wise thoughts. Moving on with his life without any animosity, or bitterness, is how he was going to live. Life was too short for animosity. He believed three factors brought him his freedom—God, the right legal team and being persistent, not giving up!

One person in commenting on Jesus' prayer wrote about having three helpful qualities—to understand, forget and love. Seek first to *understand* why people do things instead of jumping to conclusions. *"Fools find no pleasure in understanding but delight in airing their own opinions"* (Proverbs 18:2). We can *forget* in the sense that we don't let what happened control what we do today. This is what Shaurn did. *"He who covers over an offense promotes love, but whoever repeats the matter separates close friend"* (Proverbs 17:9).

Love is the third quality. This characteristic can be comparable to forgive. Paul writes, *"Love does not keep a record of wrongs"* (1 Corinthians 13:5). In other words, love forgives. Another way to think about forgiveness is to love. The poet Edwin Markham was mistreated in his life, but instead of having resentment and bitterness he practiced love. He wrote these words: "He drew a circle that shut me out—Heretic, rebel, a thing to flout. But love and I had the wit to win: We drew a circle and took him in!" When we think of forgiveness, let's practice love. Love will also release a person from stress! *"If your enemy is hungry, give him food to eat; if he is thirsty, give him water to drink"* (Proverbs 25:21).

STAYING HYDRATED PRESCRIPTION

Drink Water! *"Like a snow-cooled drink at harvest time is a trustworthy messenger to the one who sends him; he refreshes the spirit of his master."* (Proverbs 25:13). Doctor Willett of Harvard Medical School suggests drinking sixty-four ounces of water a day for a person on a 2,000-calorie meal plan.[77] Others have suggested drinking half an ounce for every pound you weigh and an ounce for every minute you exercise to keep hydrated.

French researchers discovered drinking thirty-four ounces of water per day prevented elevated blood glucose in a nine-year study of 3600 individuals.[78] The amount depends on what type of food is eaten too. Most fruits and vegetables are mainly water. Notice the water content in the following foods: fruits and vegetables (80–95%), hot cereal (85%), low-fat fruit-flavored yogurt (75%), boiled egg (75%), and fish and seafood (60–85%). When we compare a popular junk food like potato chips, we discover it has only 2 percent water content.[79] What about carbonated soft drinks? According to Doctor Willett they can work for staying hydrated, but they are loaded with sugar. And sugar-free artificially sweetened soda drinks are a concern. Many are wary of the artificial sweeteners.[80] If that is a concern, get an Infuser for fruit infused water!

A way to determine dehydration is the color of urine. Dark yellow or yellowish-brown color could indicate dehydration.[81] (Read more on drinking water in chapter eight.) "Studies have shown that being just half a litre dehydrated can increase your cortisol levels," says Amanda Carlson, RD, director of performance nutrition at Athletes' Performance, a trainer of world-class athletes. "Cortisol is one of those stress hormones. Staying in a good hydrated status can keep your stress levels down. When you don't give your body the fluids it needs, you're putting stress on it, and it's going to respond to that," says Amanda Carlson.[82] Another consideration for weight loss is to drink water. Are you really hungry or just need to drink something? Hunger may actually be the need for more fluids. How can you distinguish thirst from hunger? Sip a glass of ice water before grabbing something to eat and then wait five to ten minutes.

Thirty-six ounces of cold water a day can elevate metabolism and calorie burning by one hundred calories per day study reveals. A benefit of drinking water cold comes when drinking ice cold water. Ice cold water requires energy to warm it to core body temperature.[83]How many calories will you burn to bring an ice cold sixteen-ounce drink to body temperature? One calorie is burned for each ounce of iced beverage to warm it to core body temperature. If you were to drink sixty-four ounces a day the same number of calories would be burned! Every little bit helps![84]This is important for those with health concerns, which is all of us isn't it? Wisdom's way teaches that *"The mind of a person with understanding gets knowledge; the wise person listens to learn more"* (Proverbs 18:15 NCV).

TAKE A NAP AS YOUR ENERGY DRINK PRESCRIPTION.

**A good conscience is a soft pillow. I'm so good
at sleeping I can do it with my eyes closed.**

Taking naps has been the habit of many famous people like Albert Einstein and Winston Churchill. In fact, Winston Churchill said, "Nature has not intended mankind to work from eight in the morning until midnight without that refreshment of blessed oblivion which, even if it only lasts twenty minutes, is sufficient to renew all the vital forces." We could add more than nature, but wisdom, God's wisdom would condone taking a nap. Why? Because Jesus himself did. Remember what happened on the sea of Galilee? *"A furious squall came up, and the waves broke over the boat, so that it was nearly swamped. Jesus was in the stern, sleeping on a cushion"* (Mark 4:37-38). What is amazing about this event is that Jesus was sleeping during a storm. Have you ever had difficulty falling to sleep? All of us have, but Jesus could sleep even in the midst of a storm. How? God's wisdom gives us a key. *"Do not let wisdom and understanding out of your sight...Then you will go on your way in safety, and your foot will not stumble. When you lie down, you will not be afraid; when you lie down, your sleep will be sweet"* (Proverbs 3:22-24). *"When you walk, they will guide you; when you sleep, they will watch over you; when you awake, they will speak to you"* (Proverbs 6:22).

Have you ever had a root canal done? The procedure can be excruciating. How do you handle the pain? Meditation helps. I've gone over and over in my mind calming words like *"God is my shield and refuge"* from Proverbs 30:5. *"Every word of God is flawless; he is a shield to those who take refuge in him."* Positive wise thinking can bring a calming effect to a stressful situation. *"Be careful what you think, because your thoughts run your life"* (Proverbs 4:23 NCV). By doing this we keep in our sight wisdom and understanding, which we were told brings sweet sleep. *"Whoever seeks good finds favor, but evil comes to one who searches for it"* (Proverbs 11:27). Seek good by writing down good things that have happened during the day in your own gratitude journal.

According to a recent study, one way to remedy the negative effects of a poor night's sleep is to just take a short nap the following day. The nap was found to reduce stress and bolster the immune system. The Mayo Clinic lists the following benefits for taking naps: relaxation, reduced fatigue, increased alertness, improved mood, improved performance, including quicker reaction time and better memory. For more information about naps go to "17 Wise Ways to Outsmart Diabetes," chapter eight, number 10.

Many people aren't getting enough sleep. In fact, one in three adults report they sleep an average of six or less hours a night.[85] Drowsy driving is an ever-present danger. According to the Centers for Disease Control an estimated 1 in 25 adult drivers reports falling asleep while driving in the previous 30 days. Drowsy driving is also estimated to cause 72,000 crashes, 44,000 injuries, and 800 deaths in 2013. These numbers are underestimated and up to 6,000 fatal crashes each year may be caused by drowsy drivers.[86] For more information about sleep and getting to sleep go to "17 Wise Ways to Outsmart Diabetes," chapter nine, number 15.

17 WISE WAYS
TO OUTSMART DIABETES
ON A DAILY BASIS

CHAPTER SEVEN

Seven Wise Ways in the Morning

---

*"When you walk, they will guide you; when you
sleep, they will watch over you; when you awake,
they will speak to you"* (Proverbs 6:22).

The foundation for all of these outsmart strategies is the way of wisdom (skill for living), God's wisdom. Success and victory come from God's wisdom. *"For the LORD gives wisdom; from his mouth come knowledge and understanding. He holds success in store for the upright"* (Proverbs 2:6-7). We all have available to us God's wisdom which is more precious than rubies. *"She is more precious than rubies; nothing you desire can compare with her"* (Proverbs 3:15). The following story illustrates how we should be amazed for the rich resource God supplies, his wisdom.

MORE VALUABLE THAN RUBIES

Stunned and then overjoyed was a man when the appraised value of his blanket was revealed on the Antique Roadshow. The blanket is considered one of the Roadshow's "Greatest Finds!" The episode starts with appraiser, Donald Ellis asking the owner to tell what he knows about the blanket. He didn't know a lot except that Kit Carson was supposed to have given it to the foster father of his grandmother. He thought it was a Navajo blanket and he had never had it appraised. "Ted, did you notice that when you showed this to me I stopped breathing a little bit," said the appraiser. "It's a chief's blanket, a Ute First Phase wearing blanket. They were made from about 1840 to 1860. They were very valuable at that time. This is Navajo weaving in its purest form." Then he was told its condition is "unbelievable."

Nothing so important had been seen by him on the Roadshow. Ted did not have a clue about its value. He was then asked "are you a wealthy man?" No! An awestruck, overwhelming reaction followed when he was told its value. "On a really bad day this blanket would be worth 350,000 dollars and on a good day a half-million-dollars." Ted was astounded! If Kit Carson actually owned it he said its value would increase by 20%. Ted then became so emotional that he began to gasp for air. He was flabbergasted knowing his grandparents were just poor farmers. Some of his last words were "thank you!" Almost a half million views have been recorded of this episode on YouTube. Some of the comments are "this one really pulls on the heart strings" or "his reaction is priceless! Congratulations Sir!"

The blanket was just lying at Ted's home. We have something more valuable than rubies lying at home! What is it? Wisdom, God's word! *"Blessed are those who find wisdom, those who gain understanding.... She is more precious than rubies; nothing you desire can compare with her"* (Proverbs 3:13-15). The good news is we can use it! *"Through wisdom your days will be many, and years will be added to your life. If you are wise, your wisdom will reward you"* (Proverbs 9:11-12). This is a priceless resource that God is providing for our use! *"Trust in the LORD with all your heart and lean not on your own understanding; in all your ways acknowledge him, and he will make your paths straight"* (Proverbs 3:5-6). "Trust" is a concept that includes the idea of safety, confidence, and security. A sense of security and safety come by following God's way or wisdom. By using his wisdom life becomes straight, bringing safety, security, confidence, and better health. Learning to acknowledge God and his wisdom in a wide variety of different situations gives us hope. Yes, we have something more valuable than rubies or a Navajo Ute chief's blanket!

Watch: "Top Finds: Mid-19th Century Navajo Ute First Phase Blanket" https://www.youtube.com/watch?v=WJw2qCnhea0

So, in order to have a great day, use the following specific insights and "Way of Wisdom" principles to outsmart diabetes. Remember these proverbs from God *"are life to those who find them and health to one's whole body"* (Proverbs 4:22).

"The Road to Good Health Is Always under Construction. When You Are Through Learning, You Are Through. Keep Learning!"

"Those who cherish understanding will soon prosper" (Proverbs 19:8). *"The heart of the discerning acquires knowledge; the ears of the wise seek it out"* (Proverbs 18:15). *"A wise man has great power. A man who has knowledge increases his strength"* (Proverbs 24:5 NIrV).

17 WISE WAYS TO HAVE A GREAT DAY IN SPITE OF DIABETES!

1) The first principle is to keep learning!

Ignorance is not bliss. It is good to start the day knowing what diabetes is. The better we understand, the better our choices will be. Instead of assuming what needs to be done, we can know what needs to be done. For example, I was asked since I have Type 1 Diabetes when I would become Type 2. The fact is I will never become Type 2. Both types of diabetes have similar lifestyles with meal plans and exercise, but dissimilar with many medication treatments. The basic difference between the two is the beta cells available in the pancreas to produce insulin. Type 1 is an autoimmune disease in which the body attacks and destroys the insulin producing beta cells. Type 2 is a disease in which the cells of the body become resistant to allowing insulin, the key to opening cells for glucose and energy, to fulfill its designed function. So, it is imperative with either type to keep blood glucose as close to the normal range as possible and know that carbohydrates have a profound impact on blood glucose levels. To view an explanation of how insulin moves glucose into cells go to "Insulin, Glucose and You" at https://www.youtube.com/watch?v=jqP9JmS_sKo

For more information on what diabetes is and medications read pp. 24-25, 37-40 in my book "The Way of Wisdom for Diabetes." After knowing what diabetes is, we need to have a plan to outsmart it each day! Almost everyone has a routine in the morning, but is it best for your health?

2) The second principle is to have a health routine, a plan:

"Proper Prior Planning Prevents Pitifully Poor Performance. People Don't Plan to Fail, They Fail to Plan. Planning the Best Decisions Ahead of Time: Diligence"

"The wisdom of the prudent is to give thought to their ways, but the folly of fools is deception" (Proverbs 14:8). *"Sluggards do not plow in season; so at harvest time they look but find nothing"* (Proverbs 20:4). *"The plans of the diligent lead to profit as surely as haste leads to poverty"* (Proverbs 21:5). Biblically, the basic meaning of diligence is planning ahead. Giving thought for health is so important! How many times will I check my blood sugar today? Or how many steps will I take? How many calories will I eat and especially of carbohydrates since they directly impact my blood sugar levels? These are the things to think about first thing in the morning!

People get out of bed in the morning and usually visit the restroom. What follows among people differs. Some have the simple habit of making their bed. Making your bed first thing in the morning is good, but there is a plan that is much more beneficial for those with diabetes!

3) **The best plan, that should become a habit, is to check your blood glucose level first thing in the morning!**
   Pricking your fingers hurts! So, why do it? (Experience less pain by pricking on the side of your finger, not the pad. Use a good lancet device like a "CareTouch" too.) Discovering what your blood glucose is will give you the information to make the best decision. What if you wake up with an elevated blood glucose—185 or even 264. What should you do? Should you go ahead and eat breakfast? No, take a leisure walk instead or avoid any carbs for breakfast. What caused this? What was my blood glucose last night before going to bed? Do I have a cold starting? Did I eat a snack last night? Have relationship conflicts or financial stress? All these could be factors that cause an elevated blood glucose. Where should your blood glucose be during the day? Here are some guidelines, with a comparison to normal numbers for those without diabetes.

   - Fasting and before breakfast: 70–130 mg/dl
   - Normal is less than 100 mg/dl
   - Before lunch, supper, and snacks: 70–130 mg/dl
   - Two hours after starting meals: 160 mg/dl or less
   - Normal is less than 140 mg/dl
   - Bedtime: 90–150 mg/dl
   - Normal is less than 120 mg/dl

http://www.joslin.org/docs/Pharm_Guideline_Graded.pdf

Many people have the good habit of checking their blood glucose in the morning—and then they are through checking for the day! Research indicates that checking yourself more often than once a day will result in building greater confidence for self-management and better glucose numbers.[87] From this research the A1c test results fell more than one point—7.3 to 6.2. (For more information on this topic read pp. 31-37 in my book "The Way of Wisdom for Diabetes.)

4) **Take your medication at the right time especially if you are on insulin. The principle is the importance of timing.**

"TIMING IS (ALMOST) EVERYTHING"

Wisdom's way teaches the following on the importance of timing: *"Anyone who refuses to work doesn't plow in the right season. When he looks for a crop at harvest time, he doesn't find it"* (Proverbs 20:4 NIrV). *"Finish your outdoor work. Get your fields ready. After that, build your house"* (Proverbs 24:27). *"A person finds joy in giving an apt reply—and how good is a timely word!"* (Proverbs 15:23)

Since carbohydrates affect blood glucose be sure to take your insulin before breakfast or any meal (unless your blood glucose is below 70 then take it after the meal). Novolog and Humalog become active within fifteen to twenty minutes. So, if you wake up at 163, take your insulin, walk and then eat breakfast you could end up with a low blood glucose. This happened with a friend of mine and before he could get to breakfast he was 38 mg/dl.

5) Eat breakfast with fewer carbohydrates.

In fact, use fewer carbohydrates for every meal. Portion control is the principle.

"Wise People Keep Themselves Under Control: Portion Control, Healthy Choices, and Self-Control"

> *"If you find honey, eat just enough. If you eat too much of it, you will throw up"* (Proverbs 25:16 NIrV). *"It is not good to eat too much honey, nor does it bring you honor to brag about yourself"* (Proverbs 25:27 NCV).

Robert Buynak, MD in his book "Dr. Buynak's 1-2-3 Diabetes Diet" gives an accurate formula for determining how many calories to eat each day and maintain your current weight.[88] The formula is current weight x 11 = daily calories. For example, your weight is 230 pounds x 11 = 2500 calories per day. Since it takes 3500 calories to equal one pound, if you subtract 500 calories per day you should lose one pound per week. How many of those calories should be carbohydrates? The Joslin Diabetes Deskbook recommends 40 % of the 2000 calories as carbohydrates, that is, 800 calories (800/4 calories per gram) or 200 grams of carbohydrate per day.[89]

Since carbohydrates directly affect blood glucose levels, the less you eat the better blood glucose levels can be. What is the ideal amount of carbohydrates to eat per day? Some advocates of a low-carb meal plan really mean low-carb! Some suggest no more than 12 to 15 grams of carbs per meal which is comparable to eating just one slice of bread. For the day they suggest no more than 50 grams. Why live such a miserable life without carbs if you can eat more and still maintain blood glucose levels near normal? I usually eat about 20-25 grams for breakfast and 30-35 grams for dinner (lunch) and supper and an additional 12-15 for snacks during the day (or 110 grams per day, which equals 27 % carbs for my weight of 145 lbs.). To determine the grams of carbohydrates in various foods go to **www.calorieking.** com Using the FreeStyle Libre continuous glucose monitoring system, I've been above 140 mg/dl less than 20 % of the time with a 105-110 average.

The kind of carbohydrates to eat should be those that raise blood glucose levels least. Numbers have been assigned based on research on how fast a particular carbohydrate will make blood glucose rise in a two-hour period, compared to an equal quantity of pure glucose. All carbohydrates are compared to glucose, which is given the base line number of 100. The smaller the number is, the better the results will be for maintaining good blood glucose levels. The glycemic load (GL) number is for the "typical" serving. The result of each food can be seen by going to **www.glycemicindex.com**. The results are put into three categories, which are based on the glycemic index number. The following list has the best carbohydrates to eat with the least effect on blood glucose:

Low: 55 and under (<10 GL). Examples include:
- apple, fresh, medium (38 GI, 6 GL, 4 oz, 15 Carb grams),
- banana, fresh, medium (52 GI, 12 GL, 4 oz, 24 Carb grams)
- black beans, cooked (30 GI, 7 GL, 4/5 cup, 23 Carb grams)
- black-eyed peas, canned (42 GI, 7 GL, 2/3 cup, 17 Carb grams)
- brown rice, cooked (50 GI, 16 GL, 1 cup, 33 Carb grams),
- carrots, peeled, cooked (49 GI, 2 GL, ½ cup, 5 Carb grams)
- carrots, raw (47 GI, 3 GL, 1 medium, 6 Carb grams),
- cherries, fresh (22 GI, 3 GL, 18 cherries, 12 Carb grams),
- chickpeas or garbanzo beans, canned (42 GI, 9 GL, 2/3 cup, 22 Carb grams)
- French green beans, cooked (0 GI, 0 GL, ½ cup, 0 Carb grams)
- grapefruit, fresh, medium (25 GI, 3 GL, 1 half, 11 Carb grams)
- grapes, green, fresh (46 GI, 8 GL, ¾ cup, 18 Carb grams)
- green peas (48 GI, 3 GL, 1/3 cup, 7 Carb grams)
- honey (55 GI, 10 GL, 1 Tbsp, 18 Carb grams)
- kidney beans, canned (52 GI, 9 GL, 2/3 cup, 17 Carb grams)
- kidney beans, cooked (23 GI, 6 GL, 2/3 cup, 25 Carb grams), 28, 7)
- lentils, brown, cooked (29 GI, 5 GL, ¾ cup, 18 Carb grams)
- lentils, red, cooked, (26 GI, 5 GL, ¾ cup, 18 Carb grams)

- lima beans, baby, frozen (32 GI, 10 GL, ¾ cup 30 Carb grams)
- navy beans, canned (38 GI, 12 GL, 5 oz, 31 Carb grams)
- peach, fresh, large (42 GI, 5 GL, 4 oz, 11 Carb grams)
- peanuts (14 GI, 1 GL, 1.75 oz, 6 Carb grams)
- pear halves, canned in natural juice (43 GI, 5 GL, ½ cup, 13 Carb grams)
- pear, fresh (38 GI, 4 GL, 4 oz, 11 Carb grams)
- peas, green, frozen, cooked (48 GI, 3 GL, ½ cup, 7 Carb grams)
- pinto beans, canned (45 GI, 10 GL, 2/3 cup, 22 Carb grams)
- pinto beans, dried, cooked (39 GI, 10 GL, ¾ cup, 26 Carb grams)
- rolled oats (42 GI, 9 GL, 1 cup, 21 Carb grams)
- seeded rye bread (55 GI, 7 GL, 1 oz, 13 Carb grams)
- sourdough rye (48 GI, 6 GL, 1 oz, 12 Carb grams)
- sourdough wheat (54 GI, 8 GL, 1 oz, 14 Carb grams)
- strawberries, fresh (40 GI, 1 GL, 4 oz, 3 Carb grams)
- sweet corn, whole kernel, canned, diet-pack, drained (46 GI, 13 GL, 1 cup, 28 Carb grams)
- sweet potato, cooked (44 GI, 11 GL, 5 oz, 25 Carb grams)
- tomato, chopped (28 GI, 2 GL, 1 cup, 8 Carb grams)[90]

For a good explanation of carbohydrates watch "How do carbohydrates impact your health?"—Richard J. Wood at https://www.youtube.com/watch?v=wxzc_2c6GMg

6) Focus on staying positive every day.

One of the first things to do to start the day is to jot down good things that happened the previous day. (This could be done in the evening before going to bed as sleep preparation.) Then give thanks to God for them. Looking on the brighter side of life is the principle.

"Count Your Blessings, and You Will Show a Profit. Have the Attitude of Gratitude. Look on the Brighter Side of Life—The Good News."

"Whoever seeks good finds favor, but evil comes to one who searches for it." (Proverbs 11:27). *"A cheerful look brings joy to your heart. And good news gives health to your body"* (Proverbs 15:30). *"A cheerful heart makes you healthy. But a broken spirit dries you up"* (Proverbs 17:22 NIrV). *"Hearing good news from a land far away is like drinking cold water when you are tired"* (Proverbs 25:25 NIrV).

Health benefits from the practice of gratitude have been shown from extensive scientific research by Robert Emmons, PhD, of the University of California at Davis, by researchers at the University of Pittsburgh, University of Manchester, University of Pennsylvania and the University of Michigan and more. From this research, a practice of gratitude contributes to sleeping better, exercising more, reducing levels of the stress hormone cortisol, feeling more optimistic and connected with others. Also, people who practice gratitude have a better compliance or adherence to a meal plan and taking their medications.

Watch: "Robert Emmons: What Good is Gratitude?" at Robert Emmons: What Good Is Gratitude? https://www. youtube.com/watch?v=aRV8AhCntXc

Watch: "Yale's Most Popular Class Is Teaching Students How To Lead Happier Lives | NBC Nightly News" at https://www.youtube.com/watch?v=tarn7tJk5NE

Make sure you list the seemingly insignificant trivial things too. They shouldn't be taken for granted. We should look for minor things. Count them. List them. Pray about them. For example, we can have a good day using our hands in the yard or garden or at your computer, see the beauty of flowers and enjoy the aroma and taste of delicious food with gratitude! To see, walk, taste, feel, "eat, as well as have a home," bed, clothes, family and friends are the little things that we should appreciate and not take for granted! Watch "After Growing Up Homeless, Boy Is Over The Moon For His New Bed | NBC Nightly News" https://www.youtube.com/watch?v=vJOeC88Km-0

The following is an example of devices that directly relate to diabetes management and should be appreciated. The good news is glucose meters to check what our glucose levels are. For my first twenty-one years with diabetes, glucose meters did not even exist! Now with a very small amount of blood, glucose levels can be checked with results in five to six seconds. It hasn't always been that way! My first glucose meter was an Ames that I purchased the summer of 1981. You had to be near a sink and have a large drop of blood to use it. The blood was placed on a strip, a button would be pushed on the meter, and a one-minute countdown would start. Once a minute elapsed, a high-pressure dose of water from a small bottle was applied to the strip, washing away what blood had not absorbed into the strip. The strip was then ready to be inserted into the meter for another one-minute countdown. Finally, after following these procedures, which took over two minutes, the result would be displayed. Do you see why the Way of Wisdom principle of good news and gratitude applies to what we have available for our use today? *"A cheerful look brings joy to your heart. And good news gives health to your body"* (Proverbs 15:30 NIrV).

Now more innovative ways to check blood glucose are available—the continuous glucose monitoring systems. No finger pricks with a lancet are required. Instead a painless scan is all that is required to know what your blood glucose is. Abbott offers the user-friendly system called FreeStyle Libre. The Libre uses a scanning device called a Reader. All you have to do is place it about one inch over a sensor attached to the back of your arm. The Reader then scans from the sensor what your blood glucose level is.

The reading is from the interstitial fluid, not directly from the blood. The sensor about the size of two stacked quarters is easily attached to the back of your arm. A tiny filament remains just under the skin in the arm's interstitial fluid (We've all heard our bodies are composed of about 55-60 % fluid). Glucose first enters the blood stream before it seeps into the interstitial fluid. So, there is a short lag time between the glucose readings from continuous glucose monitoring systems and a blood glucose meter. Using the trend arrow on the reader, whether it points up or down is an indicator that your blood glucose is currently a little higher or lower than the glucose number shown. I enthusiastically recommend this devise for your use! If you are low the reader will recommend you do a blood glucose meter check. For more information go to **https://freestylelibre.us/**

If you purchase the sensors with cash, Abbot offers a cash discount card of up to almost 50 % off the list price! Go to the support section of their website and call their customer service number. Watch at Youtube "See More, Manage Better" **https://www.youtube.com/watch?v=-q8ixdYZCco&t=47s**

7) Move often throughout the day.

"Don't Just Sit There, Keep Moving"

---

*"Go to the ant, you sluggard; consider its ways and be wise! It has no commander, no overseer or ruler, yet it **stores** its provisions in summer and **gathers** its food at harvest"* (Proverbs 6:6–8). *"From the fruit of their lips people are filled with good things, and the **work of their hands** brings them reward"* (Proverbs 12:14). *"All **hard work** pays off. But if all you do is talk, you will be poor"* (Proverbs 14:23 NIrV). *"Ants are creatures of little strength, yet **they store up** their food in the summer"* (Proverbs 30:25). Keep in mind that when these proverbs were written most work involved manual labor. The principle is to move often throughout the day.

Move often is the good news for blood glucose control. Just getting up out of our chairs and leisurely walking for a couple of minutes every thirty minutes can make the difference. Research indicates that postprandial (after a meal) glucose is lowered. Not only are glucose levels reduced, but also cholesterol, triglycerides and levels of lipoprotein lipase (an enzyme that aids in the breakdown of fat in the bloodstream) are reduced.[91]

More good news comes from a study that analyzed the difference a fifteen-minute leisure walk after a meal would make on blood glucose levels compared to just sitting. Picture your blood glucose as a daunting ice-capped mountain peak by sitting compared to an image of safe, green rolling hills. By just sitting you will see your blood sugars climb higher and higher to the peak, but if walking the rise will be cut in half. So, I've learned to take a short walk after a meal rather than sit.[92]

Watch: "Have Type 2 Diabetes? Try Walking After Eating" at https://www.youtube.com/watch?v=itmdsOUVBcc

Watch: "Walk for Health: The Best Medicine" at https://www.youtube.com/watch?v=mbIM1LTfytQ

CHAPTER EIGHT

Four Wise Ways in the Afternoon

*"She (wisdom) will give you a garland to grace
your head and present you with a glorious crown.
Listen, my son, accept what I say, and the years
of your life will be many"* Proverbs 4:9-10).

8) Drink at least 34 ounces of water throughout the day.

Drink Cold Water—*"Like cold water to a weary soul is
good news from a distant land"* (Proverbs 25:25).

Remember, when reading the proverb above, the statement that is made of God's wisdom teachings in Proverbs 4:22—*"They are life to those who find them and health to one's whole body."* The basic meaning of the word *proverb* is *represent, compare,* or *be like.* Proverbs are pictures of reality. What better way to picture the gratifying, exuberant effect that good news has on a person than with the picture of the satisfaction cold water gives a really thirsty person? *"Like cold water to a weary soul is good news from a distant land"* (Proverbs 25:25).

Proverbs have more than one dimension, and the meaning here is not just about good news. In other words, the consequence of good news is pictured with the wonderful feeling that cold water gives to a thirsty person. And guess what? Cold water is good for our health.

I recently visited with a worker at a supermarket. I overheard her tell a customer how she was feeling with her diabetes. Then I had a short visit with her. She told me that she drinks water to bring down her blood glucose level which amazingly works sometimes. Why? Dehydration makes a person feel fatigued. It can also elevate the stress hormone cortisol. Cortisol is a counterregulatory hormone to insulin. Thus, when cortisol levels are elevated insulin is less effective. The result is elevated blood sugar levels. An additional way to determine dehydration is the color of urine. Dark yellow or a yellowish-brown color could indicate dehydration.[93] (Read more on Drinking Water prescription in chapter six.) "Studies have shown that being just half a litre dehydrated can increase your cortisol levels," says Amanda Carlson, RD, director of performance nutrition at Athletes' Performance, a trainer of world-class athletes. "Cortisol is one of those stress hormones. Staying in a good hydrated status can keep your stress levels down. When you don't give your body the fluids it needs, you're putting stress on it, and it's going to respond to that," says Amanda Carlson.[94] The risk of elevated blood glucose levels decreases by staying hydrated. In a nine-year study of 3,615 men and women, those who drank at least thirty-four ounces per day reduced the chances of developing elevated blood glucose problems. Those who drank more than thirty-four ounces of water per day were 21 percent less likely to develop high blood sugar than those who drank sixteen ounces or less daily. To get an accurate picture of the significance of water consumption, the analysis also took into account other factors that can affect the risk of elevated blood sugar.[95] I try to drink small amounts of water throughout the day. Six glasses with six to eight ounces of water each time. To drink it all at once isn't good for you! *"The wisdom of the prudent is to give thought to their ways"* (Proverbs 14:8).

9) **Eat healthy snacks like apples, nuts, vegetables, berries etc.**

Does An Apple a Day Keep the Doctor Away?

"Make plans by seeking advice; if you wage war, obtain guidance" (Proverbs 20:18). We all like snacks, but some snacks are unhealthy. So, to win the war against poor health we need guidance or advice to make wise choices for snacks. Knowledge is knowing a tomato or avocado is a fruit; wisdom is not putting it on a fruit salad. Knowledge is knowing donuts, donut holes, chips, pretzels, a bucket of buttered popcorn at the theater are snacks; wisdom is replacing them with healthy snacks!

What are the benefits of snacking? Snacking helps prevent overeating at meals, and it provides a constant source of nutritional fuel. Snacks help the body burn more calories, rather than storing them, by keeping the metabolic rate up. The body also gets a regular supply of fuel, which can help prevent low blood glucose levels when using insulin or sulfonylureas like Glipizide, Glimeperide, and Glyburide.

What are some good snacks to eat? Fresh fruits, like a small apple, a cup or four ounces of cherries, half of a grapefruit, twelve grapes, an orange, a peach, or a pear are good low-glycemic snacks. A popular snack is a donut hole, or should we say donut holes! A single donut hole, which weighs only half an ounce, has fifty-two calories! Whereas, 5.1 ounces of strawberries has only forty-six calories! Which one do you think will give you a more-full feeling for a snack? Low-calorie density foods, which add more volume of food to your snack are also high density nutrient snacks. One donut hole has sugar, saturated fat and flour. Whereas, the 5.1-ounce serving of strawberries has virtually no fat, but has water, three grams of fiber and anti-inflammatory antioxidants (antioxidants stop or delay damage to the cells). Strawberries have omega 3 and 6 fatty acids, minerals like magnesium, potassium and calcium and vitamins like A, C, E, K and B6.

Eat low–glycemic index carbohydrates that don't spike up blood sugars. Raw vegetables also make good snacks. Eat them with a lower-fat dip or with different flavored mustards. At our Diabetes Support Group, one person told me how she's enjoyed eating radishes and losing weight. Radishes? Yes, eating radishes. Radishes are rich in fiber, vitamin C and potassium. One cup of raw radishes has only 19 calories and 4 grams of carbohydrates. Another person said he's been eating mushrooms and has noticed better blood glucose control. Mushrooms have 23 calories for one cup with 2 grams of carbohydrates. They are also an anti-inflammatory food.

Radishes and mushrooms are much better choices than potato chips and pretzels. They are more filling. Radishes are about 90% water. Whereas, potato chips have about 2%. One serving (28 grams) of chips has 160 calories, 15 grams of carbohydrates and 10 grams of fat. One serving (28 grams) of pretzels has 100 calories and 23 grams of carbohydrates.

Deli meat wrapped in romaine lettuce leaves, low-fat cottage cheese and fruit, a boiled egg, or smoked salmon or tuna with vegetables would all be good options. Don't forget nuts like almonds, walnuts pecans and pistachios. Portion control is essential for nuts! The calories add up quickly.

Dr. Josh Axe, DNM, DC, CNS, is a certified doctor of natural medicine, doctor of chiropractic and clinical nutritionist. He lists at his website "51 Healthy Snack Ideas." His ideas with recipes include such snacks as "Baked Cinnamon Apple Chips, Five-Minute Healthy Strawberry Yogurt, Paleo Apple 'Nachos', Raw Homemade Applesauce, Very Cherry Snack Bar, Cajun Roasted Chickpeas, Zucchini Chips, Crispy Chickpea Bites, Healthy Spicy Black Bean Dip, Healthy Sweet Potato Nachos, Paprika and Chili Kale Chips, Quick Crackers, Creamy Avocado Yogurt Dip, Spiced Nuts, Roasted Pumpkin Seeds, Spicy Buffalo Cauliflower Bites and many more. Go to https://draxe.com/healthy-snack-ideas/ to read the recipes.

Watch: "Travel Foods & Snacks" at https://www.youtube.com/watch?v=F0eWaR7gJY4&t=10s

10) Eat dinner (lunch), walk and take a POWER NAP.

"I usually take a two-hour nap from one to four."—Yogi Berra

Why not take a nap? Give me one good reason? Jesus did! Remember what happened on the sea of Galilee? *"A furious squall came up, and the waves broke over the boat, so that it was nearly swamped. Jesus was in the stern, **sleeping on a cushion"** (Mark 4:37-38). When was Jesus sleeping? During a storm, yes during a storm! A wisdom insight on how he could do this is found in Proverbs 3. **"Do not let wisdom and understanding out of your sight**...Then you will go on your way in safety, and your foot will not stumble. When you lie down, you will not be afraid; when you lie down, **your sleep will be sweet"** (Proverbs 3:22-24).

Sara Mednick in her book "Take a Nap; Change Your Life" gives 20 reasons why we should take a nap.[96] Some of the reasons relate to diabetes self-management. The Ninth reason she gives is that sleepy people are more susceptible to junk food cravings.[97] The eleventh reason is to reduce your risk of diabetes or better manage it. Studies reveal sleep deprivation increases cortisol levels. Cortisol, the stress hormone causes a need for more insulin. Increased levels of cortisol bring resistance to insulin which then has a direct effect on blood glucose management.

Dr. Mednick reports that sleeplessness causes hypertension. During sleep blood pressure decreases. So, when you remain awake longer than normal, your blood pressure remains higher than normal. This can also result in a higher risk for strokes. When we deprive ourselves of sleep we enter a period of over-drive and need extra energy to support physical functions. Also, irritability, anger, depression and mental exhaustion are linked with sleeplessness. Dr. Mednick gives these guidelines for napping: keep the room as dark as possible, go for quietness and stay warm.[98]

"I usually take a two-hour nap from one to four," said Yogi Berra. What is the optimal length of time for a nap? Various lengths bring different beneficial results. If you have time to nap as long as Yogi, you would sleep through all the stages of sleep. If you don't have that kind of time even a twenty-minute nap brings benefits. Just those twenty minutes helps with rejuvenated alertness and improves motor skills like typing. Thirty to sixty-minute naps or slow-wave sleep brings better decision-making and short-term memory, but grogginess when awaking. So, during a twenty-minute power nap, which is in the lighter stages of sleep, increased energy and alertness comes when awakening. Avoid taking caffeine for up to four hours before you expect to take your nap and then your nap will become your energy drink![99]

11) Mindful Slow Eating rather than Eating in a Rush.

"It is not good to have zeal without knowledge, nor to be hasty and miss the way" (Proverbs 19:2). *"Whoever is patient has great understanding"* (Proverbs 14:29). The following is an example of how patiently eating brings about great understanding for wise mindful eating.

How do we eat? The table is set and ready for food. Twelve hungry brothers sit at the table ready to eat. Mom brings the food and sets it before them. The food is limited and these guys are famished. Can you picture the scene? The only thing you hear is the chomping of teeth. How long will it take for them to clean their plates? I can imagine asking for dessert in five minutes. When you sit down to eat you're not sitting with eleven hungry brothers are you? Yet, it is so easy to fall into the trap of devouring food without even tasting it.

Imagine a tiger chasing you. Running for your life a sharp deep cliff confronts you. You have no place to go. The tiger is getting so close you can feel him breathing down your neck, then you notice a rope dangling over the cliff and grab it. Holding onto the rope for your life, you sway, dangling from the cliff. The tiger roars above and five hundred feet below sharp jagged rocks invite you to fall. Then you notice two mice chewing on the rope above you. What should you do?

The tiger above, the rocks below and the rope is about to break! Just then you notice delicious looking bright red, ripe strawberries growing out of the side of the cliff. You stretch out one hand, pluck a strawberry and pop into your mouth. The strawberry is so sweet and refreshing. You think "Delicious— that's the best strawberry I've ever tasted."

If you were still occupied with the tiger above or the sharp rocks below you would have never tasted and enjoyed the strawberries. We call this the *precious present!* When we eat are we focusing on the smell, texture, color and rich taste of the food we're eating? Research indicates for most people the feeling of satiety (fullness) takes about twenty minutes. We haven't given ourselves time for that feeling to catch up because we're gulping down our food! So, what can we do? The Joslin Diabetes Center has a program called "Why WAIT? Weight Achievement and Intensive Treatment for Diabetes."[100] Mindful eating is taught.

Take your time. Don't get in a big hurry in eating. They suggest relaxing, taking a couple of minutes of deep breathing. Look at the food noticing its color and texture. (Pretend you will get a grade on a 500-word description you will write of the food!) Smell the food, inhaling the aroma before taking your first bite. Serve yourself less food than you think you need. Taste and savour every bite, chewing it thoroughly. To slow down your pace of eating put down your fork between each bite. Before making a decision to go back for seconds wait twenty minutes.

Watch: "Why WAIT? Weight Achievement and Intensive Treatment for Diabetes" at **https://www.youtube.com/watch?v=9r_Aw7OTZGE**

Watch: "Love to Eat? How to Eat and NOT Gain Weight" **https://www.youtube.com/watch?v=cF_zd1LxkuE**

CHAPTER NINE

Six Wise Ways In The Evening

"I instruct you in the way of wisdom and lead you along straight paths. When you walk, your steps will not be hampered; when you run, you will not stumble. Hold on to instruction, do not let it go; guard it well, for it is your life" (Proverbs 4:11-13).

12) Use tools throughout the day.

Yogi Berra on travel gear: "Why buy good luggage, you only use it when you travel."

For the best blood glucose management results use tools. Proverbs 14:4 states *"Where there are no oxen, the feed box is empty. But a strong ox brings in a great harvest."* In ancient times, oxen were essential equipment for farming (compare Deuteronomy 22:1, 10). Remember these proverbs are *"life to those who find them and health to one's whole body"* (Proverbs

4:22). The application is not oxen for our health, but tools like food scales, measuring cups, food labels, smaller plates, walking shoes that give comfort and support, a clock for timing of meds, meals and movement, record booklets or health apps and glucose meters or continuous glucose monitor systems like the FreeStyle Libre. So, good tools will equip us for better health.

One of the best tools for counting carbs in whole foods is the EatSmart™ Digital Nutrition Scale, which calculates carbs, fiber, and fats. There is a database with nutritional values for a thousand foods. For example, the number for apples is 002. After first removing the core and placing the apple on the scale, the total calories with grams of carbohydrate, and grams of fiber are given. Watch EatSmart™ Digital Nutrition Scale "Weight Loss Tool—Count Calories—EatSmart Nutrition Scale" at **https:// www.youtube.com/watch?v=AbM4Fbf9OPU**

One of the best motivational tools for getting more steps each day is a pedometer. Research was conducted with two groups wearing pedometers. The participants in one group wore a pedometer with a goal of achieving 10,000 steps a day. The other group's goal was to take a brisk, thirty-minute walk per day. The pedometers worn by the brisk, thirty-minute-a-day walking group was a non-viewable one. The group using the viewable pedometers averaged over 10,000 steps per day while the thirty-minute walking group only walked an average of 8,270 steps—a difference of almost a mile per day.

The following are comments from participants in the 2001 Diabetes in Control 10,000 step research study on the benefits of using a pedometer:

- "I reduced my stress levels."
- "It was very easy to just put on the pedometer and check it during the day—it really works."
- "I never thought I could get to ten thousand steps a day, but just by tracking my steps and increasing ten percent a week, I was able to do it!"
- "I was surprised to see that it became a habit after just a short time."
- "My whole family wanted pedometers, and they also increased their steps."
- "Just by removing the remote controllers, we picked up four hundred steps."
- "My dog is healthier than ever (I wore the pedometer, not the dog)."
- "I have more energy, and my blood sugars have never been better. Now my doctor is wearing a pedometer."
- "My blood pressure is down to normal."
- "My clothes all fit better."

The following are more beneficial tools to use.

Plate Size: "Brian Wansink, Mindless Eating" Interview concerning plate size and how the size helps with portion control at https:// www.youtube.com/watch?v=mP5AFkWZ3eY

Calorie free salad dressings: Walden Farms no calorie dressings—https:// www.waldenfarms.com/

Calculator for calories burned walking: http://calories-burnedhq.com/

Shoes: Go-Walk Skechers Shoes

Pedometers and Fitness Trackers: (They are worn on the wrist in the form of a watch. They monitor different actions like tracking daily steps, measuring heart rate and length of sleep.)

Labels: "Label Reading 101" at https://www.youtube.com/watch?v=MrdCBqFYDyo

If you were instructed to keep good records of your blood sugar readings, the amount of food you eat each day and the number of steps you take each day, would you say "You've got to be kidding"? Or "I've never done such a silly thing"? However, the way of wisdom states the concept with this principle: *"Be sure you know the condition of your flocks"* (Proverbs 27:23). Most of us do not have flocks, but we each have a body, and we need to keep track of a flock of health issues like the condition of our blood glucose levels, blood pressure, amount of sleep, exercise and movement and foods. In other words, we need to keep a daily personal health inventory. One way to do this is to keep a food diary along with records of blood glucose readings. Mynetdiary is one of many apps available. Using a tool like this helps with weight loss. In the *Journal of the American Dietetic Association*, an article titled "Food Records: A Predictor and Modifier of Weight Change in a Long-Term Weight Loss Program" concluded:

"Those who most accurately recorded their food consumption lost the most weight."[101]

Mynetdiary App., **Watch:** "MyNetDiary Overview" **https://www.youtube.com/watch?v=gVAjjkPsAY4**

13) Eat supper (dinner) earlier with less saturated fat and carbs.

"Eat Breakfast Like a King, Lunch Like a Prince, and Dinner Like a Pauper."

Wisdom's way teaches the following on the importance of timing: *"Anyone who refuses to work doesn't plow in the right season. When he looks for a crop at harvest time, he doesn't find it"* (Proverbs 20:4 NIrV). *"Finish your outdoor work. Get your fields ready. After that, build your house"* (Proverbs 24:27). *"A person finds joy in giving an apt reply—and how good is a timely word!"* (Proverbs 15:23). *"It is not good to have zeal without knowledge, nor to be hasty and miss the way"* (Proverbs 19:2).

A 20-week weight-loss treatment program was studied in Spain with 420 participants.[102] The research answered the question "Could the timing of when you eat, be just as important as what you eat?" The meal with the most calories was the lunch meal. Forty percent of daily calories were eaten for that meal. Timing of when that meal was eaten was the factor analysed to determine if the time made a difference for weight loss. Participants were divided into two groups—early eaters and late eaters. The early-eaters ate their lunch any time before 3 p.m. and late eaters, any time after 3 p.m.

Those who lost significantly less weight and at a slower rate were the late eaters group. Fewer calories for breakfast were eaten and breakfast was skipped by many. Insulin resistance also increased. "Our results indicate that late eaters displayed a slower weight-loss rate and lost significantly less weight than early eaters, suggesting that the timing of large meals could be an important factor in a weight loss program," said Frank Scheer, Ph.D., assistant professor of medicine at Harvard Medical School, and senior author on this study. Not only will eating late make it easier to gain weight, it also makes it more difficult to maintain blood sugar control. So, the lesson is to try to eat the evening meal early. The amounts of fat and carbohydrates will also determine control of blood glucose.

Someone says, "Your blood glucose is affected by sugar and carbs, so avoid them. Don't worry about other types of food!" However, wisdom's way says, *"The mind of a person with understanding gets knowledge; the wise person listens to learn more"* (Proverbs 18:15 NCV). Is fatty food just the shy, harmless guy sitting on the back row? When fatty foods are eaten, they have a powerful metabolic punch. Free fatty acids (FFAs) in the blood increase with high–saturated fat meals. What does that do? Insulin resistance increases with high–saturated fat meals. With that resistance, more insulin is needed to break through the insulin resistance barrier.

Fat also changes the timing of the rise in blood glucose after a meal. Fat takes up to six hours to move through the gastrointestinal tract. Whereas, rapid-acting insulin such as Novolog,

Humalog, or Apidra and the new Fiasp (I highly recommend because it becomes active in two minutes instead of 15 to 20 like the others) stay active for just four hours. When a high-fat meal is eaten, a significant amount of glucose still remains to be metabolized after the four-hour life of the rapid-acting insulin. This results in elevated blood glucose readings. For example, Red Robin's Bacon Cheeseburger has 71 grams of total fat with 24 being saturated. The burger also has 50 grams of carbohydrates. One effective way to combat this is get your hamburger lettuce wrapped instead with a bun and leave off the cheese.

The following is the American Heart Association's guidelines for fat consumption: Limit total fat intake to less than 25–35 percent of your total calories each day and limit saturated fat intake to less than 7 percent of total daily calories. This means that a 2000-calorie meal plan could include 140 calories from saturated fat, or 16 grams. It is also best to not eat those 16 grams all in one sitting.

Reduce consumption of saturated fats like red meat and dairy products. Think chicken, turkey, and almond milk. Monounsaturated fats like olives, avocados, cashews, almonds, peanuts, and olive and peanut oil actually lower LDL ("bad") cholesterol and insulin resistance and raise HDL. Polyunsaturated fats are found in salmon, herring, tuna, cod, pumpkin, and sunflower seeds and oil, as well as in corn oil. They also lower LDL cholesterol and triglyceride levels.[103] Instead of using canola oil which is highly processed and bitter use coconut oil, olive oil and organic butter. Dr. Axe says, "Despite unjustified warnings about saturated fat from well-meaning, albeit misinformed, experts, the list of butter's benefits is impressive: Butter is full of vitamins, minerals, and MCFA that greatly benefit overall health."[104] However, the amount used at one sitting matters for blood sugar control as previously mentioned.

Avoid meals containing 40 or more grams of fat, especially if the fat is saturated. Alter the amount and timing of your insulin if you were to eat a high-fat meal, taking an additional smaller dose later. For people with Type 2 diabetes taking oral medications, as well as those on insulin, doing some type of physical activity—for example, walking after a high-fat meal—can help control blood glucose.[105]

14) Use time restricted eating in the evening.

The study just mentioned in number 13 about 420 participants—early eaters and late eaters—also relates to this wise way. The largest meal with 40 percent of daily calories was either eaten before 3 p.m. or after. Those that benefitted most with weight loss and blood glucose control were the early eaters.

Another study at the University of Alabama called "Early Time Restricted Eating" correlates with the early eaters, late eaters research.[106] Their study of overweight people was done on two different eating schedules. One was eating from 8 am to 8 pm and the other only from 8 am to 2 pm. They discovered that more fat was burned by eating during a smaller window of time, the second category. Their research indicated, more fat was burned during the night with less food cravings during the day. I've used this idea to eat my last meal earlier in the day and especially to not eat after the last meal of the day! I maintain better blood glucose control when I can follow this schedule. (I'm not always able to do so because of my blood sugar levels getting too low before bedtime. I can't go to bed with an 80 mg/dl, especially when I know the level will drop by 30 points during most nights.) Do your own research. Try avoiding snacks during the evening and before bed. See if your blood glucose improves.

15) Have a good night's sleep.

"My son, do not let wisdom and understanding out of your sight, preserve sound judgment and discretion; they will be life for you, an ornament to grace your neck. Then you will go on your way in safety, and your foot will not stumble. When you lie down, you will not be afraid; when you lie down, your sleep will be sweet" (Proverbs 3:21-24).

Someone claims they can get by with just four or five hours of sleep per night. How many hours of sleep do we really need? The Center for Disease Control recommends, along with the Mayo Clinic, no less than seven hours a night.[107] Why? Because when we sleep we don't just dream and waste time. Our bodies are designed to use that time to stay or get healthy! Several processes are happening as we sleep. According to the National Sleep Foundation, such health benefits as "muscle repair, memory consolidation and release of hormones regulating growth and appetite" are happening.[108] This prepares us to concentrate and make decisions for all the day time activities. As we sleep, we go through five stages of sleep. These stages repeat throughout the night in about ninety-minute cycles. Our bodies are as the psalmist writes, *"Fearfully and wonderfully made"* (Psalm 139:14).

Certain foods help promote sleep. The Institute of Health Sciences recommends foods that contain tryptophan which help induce production of serotonin, which is required to make melatonin.[109] Melatonin is a hormone that regulates sleep-wake cycles. The body produces more during darkness, preparing the body for sleep. Light has the reverse affect.110

Foods that do this are grass-fed dairy products, nuts, fish, chicken, turkey, sprouted grains, beans and brown rice, eggs, sesame seeds and sunflower seeds. Eat melatonin rich foods like bananas, Morello cherries, ginger, barley, tomatoes and radishes. Include them in your dinner or supper. For a complete discussion on getting to sleep go to Dr. Josh Axe's (a certified doctor of natural medicine) article on "Top 20 Ways to Fall Asleep Fast!"[111]

16) Correct low-blood glucose: hypoglycemia.

Have Hope: A Confident Expectation That You Can Manage Diabetes. Stay Vigilant.

According to Proverbs 24:14, a person has hope when wisdom is found, inspiring a person to not give up. *"Wisdom is sweet to your soul. If you find it, there is a future hope for you, and your hope will not be cut off."* God's wisdom applies in the following way—to give thought to managing diabetes. *"The wisdom of the prudent is to give thought to their ways...The prudent see danger and take refuge"* (Proverbs 14:8, 22:3).

One of the dangers with diabetes is hypoglycemia. In the informative research I mentioned in chapter 2, the "Diabetes Attitudes, Wishes and Needs" study a deep fear of those with diabetes was discovered—hypoglycemia (blood glucose levels below 70 mg/dl).

These episodes can happen at any time during the day. So, being prudent and alert is important. Hypoglycemia is an acute stress factor for people using insulin or Sulfonylurea medications like Glipizide or Glyburide. Blood glucose can get low when too much insulin is in circulation. Counter-regulatory hormones are used to compensate for the situation. Epinephrine (commonly called adrenaline) is the "fight or flight" hormone that alerts the body to danger or stressful situations. It produces symptoms for low blood glucose like weakness, hunger, sweating, trembling, "butterflies," and heart palpitations. Epinephrine activates Glucagon. Glucagon releases stored glucose or glycogen in the liver raising blood glucose levels (glycogenolysis). A person without diabetes might experience some of these symptoms if no food has been eaten for several hours. These are the normal responses for people without diabetes, but the normal responses are compromised for those with Type 1 Diabetes or those with Type 2 on insulin or medications like Glipizide because too much insulin may be in circulation. So, taking carbohydrates to raise the blood sugar level is important to prevent dangerous lows.

The epinephrine response gets blunted for many people who have had Type 1 diabetes a long time. They lose the early warning signs of low blood glucose. Lower and lower blood glucose levels have to occur before its response occurs. So, instead of being in the 60's mg/dl blood glucose levels it may be less than 40 mg/dl. According to the Joslin Diabetes Center, new research indicates that avoidance of hypoglycemia episodes can restore the proper timely response of the epinephrine, giving the warning signs at a much higher safer blood glucose level.[112] A great precaution we can take is to check our blood glucose more often. When I'm not using my Freestyle Libre continuous glucose monitoring system, I'm checking myself up to twelve times a day. The practice of checking yourself often is important especially if you are on insulin or the medications previously mentioned. This reduces the risk of having a severe episode! Another precaution is to have glucose tablets or Smarties™ or SweeTarts™ with you at all times. For a visual episode of not taking this precaution while on a walk watch "Jim's 1st Person Low" at https://www.youtube.com/watch?v=f7SEaZSWqXs

How many grams of a quick-energy carbohydrate are needed to treat a low reading of blood glucose? A good rule of thumb is that 1 gram of glucose raises the blood sugar 3, 4, or 5 points for body weights of 200, 150, or 100 pounds, respectively. For example, 5 grams of dextrose, as found in Smarties™ or SweeTarts™ raises the blood sugar about 20 points for a 150-lb person.[113]

Treat a low with 15 grams of Smarties™ or similar candy, then wait twenty minutes and check again. Also, use a combination of a low glycemic index carbohydrate with a fast-acting carbohydrate. For example, I woke up one night about 2 am to visit the restroom. I decided to check my blood glucose and discovered it was 46 mg/dl. So, I took 9 grams of Smarties™ (GI of 96) and a small amount of milk (6 grams of carb—GI of 34). When I checked my blood glucose at 6 am I was 116. Since I weigh about 150 lbs. the 15 grams of carb should have elevated my blood glucose by 60 points. That number and combination of carbs brought my blood glucose level up by 70 points. Measuring the amount of carbohydrates will prevent overcompensating and ending up with a high blood glucose! This plan has worked for me in the almost sixty years I've had diabetes, preventing ambulance calls and hospitalization.

17) Take advantage of opportunities to help others.

To Be Encouraged, Encourage

"A good person gives life to others; the wise person teaches others how to live" (Proverbs 11:30).

Glenn lived by himself (He had LADA diabetes for twenty years—Latent Autoimmune Diabetes in Adults, a progressively slow developing Type 1 with his beta producing insulin cells are being destroyed). He picked up a diabetes support group business card at the local pharmacy. He started attending the meetings. He gave encouragement and received support from others who were also facing many of the same challenges with diabetes.

"A generous person will prosper; whoever refreshes others will be refreshed" (Proverbs 11:25). This wisdom was put into practice by him. He became very involved with the community diabetes support group. When several of us would meet to count advertising flyers for a diabetes seminar to mail, he would be there! He knew that people would attend and be helped because of one of many flyers he counted to be mailed. He would set up chairs in the large community room at the library for seminar participants. He was helping, being encouraged and encouraging!

Blood glucose control was a perpetual struggle for him. God has designed the human body in a marvellous way. When carbohydrates are eaten and they reach the small intestine, a hormone (GLP1), a messenger goes to the pancreas and signals for an initial release of stored insulin and the manufacturing of more. The amount is exact to meet the needs of the amount of carbohydrates eaten. The blood glucose will be kept in a tight range usually between 70 to 140 mg/dl. But people like Glenn do not have the beta cells that produce the insulin. They've been destroyed. He required a strict balancing act, which is a great challenge! It's been said that managing diabetes is like playing the piano with your right hand while you are juggling with your left hand all while trying to keep your balance as you walk on a tightrope. Managing diabetes is a balancing act!

All Glenn had to do was take his insulin at the right time, in just the right amount, several times each day; check his blood sugars multiple times a day to make sure he wasn't too high or too low; balance the right amount of food with the insulin he took. Stay alert at all times for stress or colds which elevate the stress hormone cortisol causing elevated blood sugars. And also realize this must be done every day, because there is never a vacation from diabetes. That's how simple it can be! People like Glenn need encouragement! We all need to give help and receive help!

There is nothing like experiencing a low, low blood sugar. In a sense, a very low reading is like trying to squeeze out every ounce or milligram of glucose to just stay conscious. Glenn's blood glucose was a rollercoaster of ups and downs. I called him one afternoon asking how he was doing. He was out of blood glucose checking strips. He had been having lows and some were very, very low. I told him my wife and I would bring him some strips. We found him on his bedroom floor, helpless, sitting with his legs crossed in his briefs. His eyes were glazed. He barely recognized me.

Immediately I checked his blood glucose. It was 20 mg/dl. This was a severe hypoglycemic episode. The race was on to keep him conscious. Since he was awake and could swallow I gave him Smarties™ from my own glucose checking kit. The Smarties™ eventually brought him out of the severe low. Ten days later he had another severe episode. No one was there to help and he passed away. There are many people who need a helping hand. I've had many who have helped me—my wife, parents, friends, doctors and nurses. Each day let's think about helping others.

God's wisdom applies in the following way—to give thought to what we do. *"The wisdom of the prudent is to give thought to their ways...The prudent see danger and take refuge"* (Proverbs 14:8, 22:3). A great precaution we all can take is to check our blood glucose more often. The other practice is to keep focused on helping others. Not only will they benefit, but we will too!

In conclusion, many of us can relate to the following story. Let's use the lessons in this story to help others in their lives and ours and with health concerns. When we do, we will all benefit! Let's support others!

"Two are better than one, because they have a good return for their labor: If either of them falls down, one can help the other up. But pity anyone who falls and has no one to help them up" (Ecclesiastes 4:9-10).

Remember when you were in school. Were you comfortable sitting with your friends at lunchtime? Or, do you remember lunchtime being a time you dreaded because you sat alone? Sitting by yourself is lonely and uncomfortable especially when everyone else seems to be laughing and enjoying the company of friends. How many new kids sitting alone may think they are being the objects of the laughter?

Long ago I heard a professor share this interesting saying: "It's not what I think that's important; it's not what you think that is important, but it's what I think you think that's important." There are usually no lunchtime welcoming committees for new kids! Most students or teenagers show little concern about new people. *"A person who isn't friendly looks out only for himself"* (Proverbs 18:1). How true that proverb is at lunchtime in many schools.

At Boca High School in Florida the whole lunch-time scenario was abruptly halted by a group called "We Dine Together." Denis Estimon and three other students began the year with a determination to not let anyone eat alone unless they wanted to. This started during Denis's senior year, but he remembered being lonely as an immigrant back when he was a first grader. Dozens are now members out of a high school of 3,400 students. Other schools have initiated "We Dine Together" clubs. Comments of appreciation for these acts of kindness are often expressed by people in their 50's who also remember how it was. Their comments were like "lunch periods were achingly uncomfortable" or "I walked instead of ate lunch." One mother discovered her son suffered from social isolation so much that he would hide while he ate.

What would Jesus do? He taught *"Do to others as you would have them do to you"* (Luke 6:31). Jesus reached out to people who were socially isolated—lepers, tax collectors, the sick. He even ate with tax collectors who were avoided and ridiculed by others. Jesus knew kindness and attention is greatly appreciated. *"Always try to be kind to each other and to everyone else...clothe yourselves with compassion, kindness, humility, gentleness and patience...whoever refreshes others will be refreshed...goodwill is found among the upright"* (1 Thessalonians 5:15, Colossians 3:12, Proverbs 11:25, 14:9).

These teenagers are practicing God's wisdom in a wonderfully kind way! "We Dine Together" clubs are running in 15 other schools now with 100 more scheduled to start.

Watch: "So no student eats alone" at https://www.youtube.com/watch?v=IfIl5Rw6dBQ and https://www.facebook.com/wedinetogether/

Let's not let others suffer alone. Let's support others because God is supporting us with his wisdom. God, through his wisdom is giving us great power to overcome, be resilient and persevere! *"The wise prevail through great power, and those who have knowledge muster their strength...For the LORD gives wisdom; from his mouth come knowledge and understanding. He holds success in store for the upright...Do not let them out of your sight, keep them within your heart; for they are life to those who find them and health to one's whole body"* (Proverbs 24:5, 2:7-8, 4:21-22).

About the Authors

KEN ELLIS is a survivor of diabetes for almost sixty years, being diagnosed when he was in the first grade during the fall of 1960. For more than twenty-five years he has facilitated hospital and community diabetes support groups, helping hundreds of people to manage their diabetes in several states.

Ken has participated in the 50-year medalist research study and has been awarded the 50-Year Medal from the world-renowned Joslin Diabetes Center, which is affiliated with Harvard Medical School in Boston. This award represents his accomplishment of diabetes management for fifty years.

DEB ELLIS is a skilled secretary. She is experienced in Corporate, Government and School Administration secretarial responsibilities. More importantly, she is Ken's wife for more than forty years, helping him with meal planning and giving positive support for his diabetes management!

KEN'S EDUCATION: Degree of Master of Science in Biblical Studies, Abilene Christian University, 1982
Contact: www.wisdomfordiabetes.org
email: ken@wisdomfordiabetes.org

Subscribe to the "Wisdom, Good News, Health and Wellness" newsletter at www.wisdomfordiabetes.org

Bible Versions

Endnotes

Introduction: The Power of Wisdom

1   http://www.newson6.com/story/21480244/tahlequah-wwii-vet-touches-lives-with-battle-agasint-illiteracy (Accessed October 18, 2016).

2   http://diatribe.org/medtronics-minimed-670g-hybrid-closed-loop-trial-ending-month (Accessed October 18, 2016).

3   http://hsci.harvard.edu/news/stem-cells-billions-human-insulin-producing-cells (Accessed October 18, 2016).

4   Brian Wansink, Slim by Design: Mindless Eating Solutions for Everyday Life (New York: HarperCollins, 2014) Kindle Locations 697-700.

5   Virgil M. Fry, Rekindled: Warmed by Fires of Hope (Abilene, Texas: Leafwood Publishers, 2007), 72-73.

6   https://www.cbsnews.com/news/teen-shark-attack-survivor-recalls-harrowing-attack-in-north-carolina/ (Accessed May 4, 2018).

7   http://wlns.com/2016/06/10/a-teen-a-puppy-and-a-wish-granted/ (Accessed May 4, 2018)

8   Hundreds repaint older man's home after teens make hurtful comments, Mary Bowerman, https://www.usatoday.com/story/news/nation-now2015/08/11/oregon-railroad-worker-elderly-neighbor-good-samaritan-paint/31458297/ (Accessed May, 2018).

Chapter 1 - The Power of Optimism

9   Norman Cousins, Anatomy of an Illness as Perceived by the Patient: Reflections on Healing and Regeneration (Kindle Location 57). Open Road Media. Kindle Edition.

10 Norman Cousins, Anatomy of an Illness as Perceived by the Patient (Kindle Location 109).

11 Robert Tattersall. Diabetes: The Biography (Biographies of Disease). Oxford University Press. Kindle Edition.

12 Norman Cousins. Anatomy of an Illness as Perceived by the Patient (Kindle Location 241).

13 Norman Cousins, Head First: The Biology of Hope (New York: E.P. Dutton, 1989), 80-81, 87

14 Personal Accounts of the Negative and Adaptive Psychosocial Experiences of People With Diabetes in the Second Diabetes Attitudes, Wishes and Needs (DAWN2) Study, Heather L. Stuckey, Diabetes Care September, 2014 http://care.diabetesjournals.org/content/37/9/2466 (Accessed May, 2018).

15 Second Diabetes Attitudes, Wishes and Needs (DAWN2) Study, Heather L. Stuckey.

16 Robert A. Emmons, Thanks: How Practicing Gratitude Can Make You Happier (New York: Houghton Mifflin Company, 2007), 27. Emmons, 32–33.

17 Stephen Post, Why Good Things Happen to Good People: The Exciting New Research That Proves the Link Between Doing Good and Living a Longer, Healthier, Happier Life (New York: Broadway Books, 2007), 28, 30.

18   Personal Health, Jane E. Brody, **http://www.nytimes. com/1988/04/07/us/health-personal-health.html** (Accessed May, 2018.

19   Is Laughter The Best Medicine?, R. Morgan Griffin, WebMD April 7, 2006 **http://www.cbsnews.com/news/is-laughter-the-best-medicine/2/** (Accessed May, 2018).

20   A good sense of humor is a sign of psychological health, Janet M. Gibson, **https://qz.com/768622/a-good-sense-of-humor-is-a-sign-of-psychological-health/** (Accessed May, 2018).

21   Grin and bear it: the influence of manipulated facial expression on the stress response, **https://www.ncbi.nlm. nih.gov/pubmed/23012270** (accessed April, 2017).

22   Does Singing Make You Happy?, Julia Layton, **http:// science.howstuffworks.com/life/inside-the-mind/emotions/ singing-happy1.htm** (Accessed May, 2018).

23   Singing Changes Your Brain, Stacy Horn, August 16, 2013, **http://ideas.time.com/2013/08/16/singing-changes-your-brain/** (Accessed May, 2018)

24   11 Surprising Health Benefits of Singing, **http:// takelessons.com/blog/health-benefits-of-singing** (Accessed May, 2018).

Chapter 2 – The Power of Kindness

25   Toddler 'Running Down' Busy Oregon Highway Caught on Dashcam Video, Avianne Tan, January 22, 2016, **https:// abcnews.go.com/US/toddler-running-busy-oregon-highway-caught-dashcam-video/story?id=36447277** (Accessed May, 2018).

26   Ants and Survival Rafts, John Clayton, **http://www. doesgodexist.org/JanFeb14/AntsandSurvivalRafts-DD.html**

27   Boston driver returns homeless man's $187,000 inheritance left in taxi, Ashley May, USA TODAY, July 6, 2016 **https://www.usatoday.com/story/news/nation-now/2016/07/06/boston-driver-returns-homeless-mans-187000-inheritance-left-taxi/86742594/** (Accessed May, 2018).

28   College Student, 24, Pays Off Grandparents' Mortgage by Saving Money Eating Microwave Pizza and Skipping Parties, Naja Rayne, Peoplecelebrity, March 26, 2016, **http://people.com/celebrity/houston-college-student-pays-off-grandparents-mortgage/** (Accessed May, 2018).

29   California man dies after paying stranger's $200 grocery bill, inspiring her to pay it forward, Alexandra Zaslow, Today, December 2, 2015 **https://www.today.com/news/california-man-dies-after-paying-strangers-200-grocery-bill-inspiring-t59206** (Accessed May, 2018).

30   College Prof Babysits Single Mom's Kids So That She Can Take Final Exam, Josh Starling, Inspiremore, December 14, 2015, **https://www.inspiremore.com/college-professor-babysits-moms-kids-while-she-takes-final/** (Accessed May, 2018).

31   'I had to do something': Repo man raises money to save elderly couple's car, Rheana Murray, Today, November 23, 2016, **https://www.today.com/kindness/illinois-repo-man-jim-ford-raises-money-save-elderly-couple-t105271** (Accessed May, 2018).

32   Viral photo shows Chick-fil-A employee continuing to work through injury, Patrick Tolbert, Kxan, December 15, 2016, http://www.kxan.com/news/national-news/viral-photo-shows-chick-fil-a-employee-continuing-to-work-through-injury/995038316 (Accessed May, 2018).

33   Frankfort employee gives a gift of life, Susan DeMar Lafferty, Chicago Tribune, March 2, 2015, http://www.chicagotribune.com/news/local/breaking/ct-sta-frankfort-transplant-st-0303-20150302-story.html (Accessed May, 2018).

34   Good Samaritan takes off boots, gives them to homeless man on CTA train, Sarah Schulte, Chicago WLS, Monday, January 15, 2018, http://abc7chicago.com/society/good-samaritan-gives-homeless-man-shoes-off-his-feet/2946604/ (Accessed May, 2018).

35   Volunteering may be good for body and mind, Stephanie Watson, Harvard Health Publishing, http://www.health.harvard.edu/blog/volunteering-may-be-good-for-body-and-mind-201306266428 (Accessed May, 2018).

36   Helping people, changing lives: The 6 health benefits of volunteering, http://mayoclinichealthsystem.org/hometown-health/speaking-of-health/helping-people-changing-lives-the-6-health-benefits-of-volunteering (Accessed May, 2018).

37   Random Acts of Kindness, https://www.randomactsofkindness.org/kindness-ideas (Accessed May, 2018).

38   Metro Rescue Victim To Become Firefighter, Christy Lewis, Oklahoma City News9, February 23, 2018, http://www. news9.com/story/37580818/metro-rescue-victim-to-become-firefighter (Accessed May, 2018).

Chapter 3 – The Power of Motivation

39   Woman drops 40 pounds so she can donate her kidney to ailing friend, Chloe Aiello, Today, May 19, 2017, https:// www.today.com/health/woman-drops-40-pounds-so-she-can-donate-her-kidney-t111598 (Accessed May, 2018).

40   Meet Quasimodo, a Dog With Rare Short Spine Syndrome Who is Thriving, Aly Semigran, PetMD, February 04, 2016, https://www.petmd.com/news/lifestyle-entertainment/ what-short-spine-syndrome-rare-congenital-disorder-found-hound-dogs-335-33510 (Accessed May, 2018).

41   Meet Florence 'See See' Rigney, America's 'Oldest Working Registered Nurse', David Douglas and Catie Beck, NBC News, March 22, 2017, https://www.nbcnews.com/nightly-news/meet-florence-see-see-rigney-america-s-oldest-working-nurse-n737451 (Accessed May, 2018).

42   Robert A. Emmons, Thanks: How Practicing Gratitude Can Make You Happier (New York: Houghton Mifflin Company, 2007), 27. Emmons, 32– 33.

Chapter 4 – The Power of Movement

43   World's longest running streak ends at 19,032 days, Lenny Bernstein, Washington Post, January 30, 2017, http://www. chicagotribune.com/sports/international/ct-longest-running-streak-spt-20170130-story.html (Accessed May, 2018).

44 This 92-year-old just became the oldest woman to run a marathon, Cindy Boren, Washington Post, May 31, 2015, https://www.washingtonpost.com/news/early-lead/wp/2015/05/31/harriette-thompson-92-is-trying-to-become-oldest-woman-to-run-a-marathon/?noredirect=on&utm_term=.324441d9ff3e (Accessed May, 2018).

45 WWII veteran Ernie Andrus turns 93, finishes coast-to-coast run on schedule, Michelle Matthews, Real-Time News from Mobile, August 20, 2016, https://www.al.com/news/mobile/index.ssf/2016/08/wwii_veteran_ernie_andrus_turn.html (Accessed May, 2018).

46 Plano Man Walks 15 Miles to Work in McKinney Every Day, Homa Bash, NBCDFW 5, February 19, 2017, https://www.nbcdfw.com/news/local/Plano-Man-Walks-15-Miles-to-Work-in-McKinney-Every-Day-414213643.html (Accessed May, 2018).

47 Standing for healthier lives—literally, Francisco Lopez-Jimenez, MD, Mayo Clinic. https://academic.oup.com/eurheartj/article/36/39/2650/2398350 (Accessed May, 2018).

48 Stand up, sit less and move more, researchers say; here's how to do it, Carina Storrs, CNN August 6, 2015, http://www.cnn.com/2015/08/06/health/how-to-move-more/index.html (Accessed May, 2018).

49 New CDC report: More than 100 million Americans have diabetes or prediabetes, July 18, 2017, https://www.cdc.gov/media/releases/2017/p0718-diabetes-report.html (Accessed May, 2018).

50   The Origin of the 10,000-Steps-Per-Day Goal, Natalie Shoemaker, http://bigthink.com/ideafeed/the-origin-of-the-10000-steps-per-day-goal (Accessed May, 2018).

51   The Surprising Number of Steps Americans Really Take Each Day, Sarah Klein, Health, July 13, 2017, http://www.health.com/fitness/number-of-steps-americans-take-daily (Accessed May, 2018).

52   Adult Obesity Facts, https://www.cdc.gov/obesity/data/adult.html (Accessed May, 2018).

53   Walking, https://www.cdc.gov/physicalactivity/walking/index.htm (Accessed May, 2018).

54   How Many Steps/Day Are Enough? Preliminary Pedometer Indices for Public Health, Catrine Tudor-Locke, PhD, and David R. Bassett, Jr., PhD, https://www.renevanmaarsseveen.nl/wp-content/uploads/overig6/how%20many%20steps%20are%20enough%20-%20catrine%20tudor%20locke.pdf (Accessed May, 2018).

55   Walking 10,000 steps/day or more reduces blood pressure and sympathetic nerve activity in mild essential hypertension. https://www.ncbi.nlm.nih.gov/pubmed/11131268 (Accessed May, 2018).

56   Increasing daily walking improves glucose tolerance in overweight women. https://www.ncbi.nlm.nih.gov/pubmed/14507493 (Accessed May, 2018).

Chapter 5 – The Power of Nutrition

57   Portion Distortion, https://www.nhlbi.nih.gov/health/educational/wecan/eat-right/portion-distortion.htm (Accessed May, 2018).

58   Break the Cycle of Yo-Yo Dieting, Jennifer Hubert, DO, St. Joseph Health Medical Group, January 9, 2018, https://www.stjhs.org/healthcalling/2018/january/break-the-cycle-of-yo-yo-dieting/ (Accessed May, 2018).

59   100-Year-Old Woman Breaks World Record at Penn Relays, Carly Hoilman, The Blaze, May 1, 2016, https://www.theblaze.com/news/2016/05/01/100-year-old-woman-breaks-world-record-at-penn-relays (Accessed May, 2018).

60   Energy density and weight loss: Feel full on fewer calories, Mayo Clinic Staff, http://www.mayoclinic.com/health/weight-loss/NU00195 (Accessed May, 2018).

61   Josh Axe, The Real Food Diet Cookbook: delicious real recipes for losing weight, feeling great, and transforming your health (Nashville: Exodus Health Center LLC. Kindle Edition, 2011), Kindle Locations 241-242.

62   Nutrition and healthy eating, Mayo Clinic Staff, https://www.mayoclinic.org/healthy-lifestyle/nutrition-and-healthy-eating/in-depth/dietary-guidelines/art-20045584 (Accessed May, 2018).

63   Richard Beaser, MD, ed., Joslin Diabetes Deskbook: A Guide for Primary Care Providers (Boston: Joslin Diabetes Center, 2014), 110.

64   Improving Your Health with Fiber, The Cleveland Clinic, http://my.clevelandclinic.org/healthy_living/nutrition/hic_improving_your_health_with_fiber.aspx (Accessed May, 2018).

65   Fiber Content of Foods in Common Portions Harvard University Health Services, **http://huhs.harvard.edu/ assets/File/OurServices/Service_Nutrition_Fiber.pdf** (Accessed May, 2018).

66   Barbara Rolls, PhD, The Volumetrics Eating Plan: Techniques and Recipes for Feeling Full on Fewer Calories (New York: HarperCollins Publishers, 2005), 10.

67   Calorie Density Key To Losing Weight, Penn State June 8, 2007, ScienceDaily. **http://www.sciencedaily.com/ releases/2007/06/070608093819.htm** (Accessed May, 2018).

68   Police make unusual withdrawal from ATM - a man stuck inside, Sarah Coles, Aol, July 14, 2018, **https://www.aol. co.uk/news/2017/07/14/police-make-unusual-withdrawal-from-atm-a-man-stuck-inside/** (Accessed May, 2018).

69   Salad and Satiety: Energy Density and Portion Size of a First-Course Salad Affect Energy Intake at Lunch, Barbara Rolls, PhD, Department of Nutritional Sciences, Pennsylvania State University, October, 2004 **http://www. ncbi.nlm.nih.gov/pubmed/15389416** (Accessed May, 2018).

70   Romaine Lettuce Nutrition, Benefits & Recipes, Dr. Axe, **https://draxe.com/romaine-lettuce-nutrition/** (Accessed May, 2018).

Chapter 6 – The Power of Stress Control

71   Gary Arsham, MD, and Ernest Lowe, Diabetes: A Guide to Living Well (Alexandria, Virginia: American Diabetes Association, 2004), 183-184.

72 Joseph P. Napora, PhD, Stress-Free Diabetes: Your Guide to Health and Happiness (Alexandria, Virginia: American Diabetes Association, 2010), 1–2.

73 Virgil M. Fry, Rekindled: Warmed by Fires of Hope (Abilene, Texas: Leafwood Publishers, 2007), 72-73.

74 5-Year-Old Alabama Boy's Act of Kindness Moves Homeless Man, Restaurant Patrons to Tears, Tracy Bloom, KTLA 5, May 19, 2015, **http://ktla.com/2015/05/19/5-year-old-alabama-boys-touching-gesture-moves-homeless-man-to-tears/** (Accessed May, 2018).

75 Praying for Others, Financial Strain, and Physical Health Status in Late Life, Neal Krause, Journal for the Scientific Study of Religion, Vol. 42, No. 3 (Sep., 2003), pp. 377-391 **http://www.jstor.org/stable/1387741?seq=1#page_scan_tab_contents** (Accessed May, 2018).

76 Wrongfully Convicted Man Holds No Grudge after Spending 24 Years in Prison, McKinley Corbley, Good News Network, May 27, 2017, **https://www.goodnewsnetwork.org/wrongfully-convicted-man-holds-no-grudge-spending-24-years-prison-feel-wonderful/** (Accessed May, 2018).

77 Walter Willett, MD, Eat, Drink, and Weigh Less: A Flexible and Delicious Way to Shrink your Waist Without Going Hungry (New York: Tante Malka, Inc., 2006), 67.

78 Drinking Water May Cut Risk of High Blood Sugar, Charlene Laino, **http://diabetes.webmd.com/news/20110630/drinking-water-may-cut-risk-of-high-blood-sugar** (Accessed March 12, 2018).

79   Barbara Rolls, PhD, The Volumetrics Eating Plan: Techniques and Recipes for Feeling Full on Fewer Calories (New York: HarperCollins Publishers, 2005), 10.

80   Artificial sweeteners: sugar-free, but at what cost?, Holly Strawbridge **https://www.health.harvard.edu/ blog/artificial-sweeteners-sugar-free-but-at-what-cost-201207165030** (Accessed March 16, 2018).

81   Urine Color, Mayo Clinic Staff, **https://www.mayoclinic.org/ diseases-conditions/urine-color/symptoms-causes/syc-20367333** (Accessed March 12, 2018)

82   Water and Stress Reduction: Sipping Stress Away, Gina Shaw, **http://www.webmd.com/diet/features/water-stress-reduction** (Accessed March 12, 2018).

83   Robert K. Cooper, PhD, Flip the Switch Lose the Weight: Proven Strategies to Fuel Your Metabolism & Burn Fat 24 Hours a Day (New York: Rodale Inc., 2005), 78-79.

84   Brian Wansink, PhD, Mindless Eating: Why We Eat More Than We Think (New York: Bantam Dell, 2006), 189.

85   The Health Benefits of Napping: Resting Can Help Reduce Stress and Protect Immune System, Lecia Bushak, Medical Daily, February 10, 2015, **http://www.medicaldaily.com/ health-benefits-napping-resting-can-help-reduce-stress-and-protect-immune-system-321580** (Accessed May, 2018).

86   Drowsy Driving: Asleep at the Wheel, **https://www.cdc. gov/features/dsdrowsydriving/index.html** (Accessed April, 2018).

Chapter 7 – Seven Wise Ways in the Morning

87 American Association of Diabetes Educators: People with Type 2 Diabetes Do Indeed Benefit From Blood Glucose Self-Monitoring: Study, August, 2015, http://www. newswise.com/articles/people-with-type-2-diabetes-do-indeed-benefit-from-blood-glucose-self-monitoring-study (Accessed May, 2018).

88 Robert Buynak, MD, Dr. Buynak's 1-2-3 Diabetes Diet: A Step-by-Step Approach to Weight Loss without Gimmicks or Risks (Alexandria, Virginia: American Diabetes Association, 2006), 13, 85.

89 Richard Beaser, MD, ed., Joslin Diabetes Deskbook: A Guide for Primary Care Providers (Boston: Joslin Diabetes Center, 2014), 93.

90 Jennie Brand-Miller, PhD, Kaye Foster-Powell, and Rick Mendosa, What Makes My Blood Glucose Go Up . . . and Down?: And 101 Other Frequently Asked Questions About Your Blood Glucose Levels (New York: Marlowe & Company, 2003), 173-182.

91 Breaking Up Prolonged Sitting Reduces Postprandial Glucose and Insulin Responses, http://care. diabetesjournals.org/content/35/5/976 (Accessed May, 2018).

92 James A. Levine, Get Up!: Why Your Chair is Killing You and What You Can Do About It, (St. Martin's Press. Kindle Edition), 68-69.

Chapter 8 – Four Wise Ways in the Afternoon

93 Urine Color, https://www.mayoclinic.org/diseases-conditions/urine-color/symptoms-causes/syc-20367333 (Accessed March 12, 2018).

94 Water and Stress Reduction: Sipping Stress Away, Gina Shaw, http://www.webmd.com/diet/features/water-stress-reduction (Accessed March 12, 2018).

95 Drinking Water May Cut Risk of High Blood Sugar, Charlene Laino, http://diabetes.webmd.com/news/20110630/drinking-water-may-cut-risk-of-high-blood-sugar (Accessed March 12, 2018).

96 Sara C. Mednick, PhD, Mark Ehrman, Take a Nap! Change Your Life, (New York: Workman Publishing Company. Kindle Edition, 2006), 23.

97 Sleep Deprivation Linked To Junk Food Cravings, Stephanie Castillo, February 29, 2016, http://www.medicaldaily.com/sleep-deprivation-weight-gain-munchies-375684 (Accessed March 22, 2018).

98 Sara C. Mednick, PhD, Mark Ehrman, Take a Nap! Change Your Life, (New York: Workman Publishing Company. Kindle Edition, 2006), 88.

99 How Long is an Ideal Nap? https://sleep.org/articles/how-long-to-nap/ (Accessed May, 2018).

100 Osama Hamdy, Sheri R. Colberg, The Diabetes Breakthrough: Based on a Scientifically Proven Plan to Lose Weight and Cut Medications (Onario: Harlequin Enterprises Limited, 2013), Kindle Locations 2952-2954.

Chapter 9 – Six Wise Ways in the Evening

101   Robert K. Cooper, PhD, Flip the Switch Lose the Weight: Proven Strategies to Fuel Your Metabolism & Burn Fat 24 hours A Day (New York: Rodale Books, 2005), 144.

102   Could the Timing of When You Eat, Be Just as Important as What You Eat?, Science Daily, January 29, 2013, http://www.sciencedaily.com/releases/2013/01/130129080620.htm (Accessed May, 2018).

103   Lucy Beale, RD, CDE, and Joan Clark, RD, CDE, Glycemic Index Weight Loss: Easy-to-Follow Diet Plans That Keep Your Weight Low and Metabolism High (New York: Penguin Group, 2005), 116–18.

104   Josh Axe, The Real Food Diet Cookbook: delicious real recipes for losing weight, feeling great, and transforming your health, (Nashville: Exodus Health Center LLC. Kindle Edition, 2011), Kindle Locations 486-488.

105   Joslin Communications, Why Does Fat Increase Blood Glucose? http://blog.joslin.org/2011/09/why-does-fat-increase-blood-glucose/#.TqadrIVmud4.email (Accessed May, 2018).

106   Time-restricted feeding study shows promise in helping people shed body fat, Adam Pope, January 09, 2017, https://www.uab.edu/news/health/item/7869-time-restricted-feeding-study-shows-promise-in-helping-people-shed-body-fat (Accessed May, 2018).

107   How Much Sleep Do I Need?, https://www.cdc.gov/sleep/about_sleep/how_much_sleep.html (Accessed June, 2018).

108 What Happens When You Sleep?, **https://sleepfoundation. org/how-sleep-works/what-happens-when-you-sleep/ page/0/1** (Accessed June, 2018).

109 Maximising Your Melatonin, **https:// instituteofhealthsciences.com/maximising-your-melatonin/** (Accessed June, 2018).

110 Melatonin, **https://www.webmd.com/vitamins/ai/ ingredientmono-940/melatonin** (Accessed June, 2018).

111 Top 20 Ways to Fall Asleep Fast! Dr. Josh Axe, **https:// draxe.com/cant-sleep/** (Accessed June, 2018).

112 Richard Beaser, MD, ed., Joslin Diabetes Deskbook: A Guide for Primary Care Providers (Boston: Joslin Diabetes Center, 2014), 437-440.

113 John Walsh, PA, CDE, Using Insulin: Everything You Need for Success with Insulin (San Diego: Torrey Pines Press, 2003), 220.

www.ingramcontent.com/pod-product-compliance
Lightning Source LLC
Chambersburg PA
CBHW072120020426
42334CB00018B/1662